COLOR & HUMAN RESPONSE

**Aspects of light and color bearing on
the reactions of living things and
the welfare of human beings**

FABER BIRREN

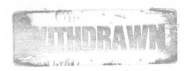
VNR **VAN NOSTRAND REINHOLD COMPANY**
New York   Cincinnati   Toronto   London   Melbourne

The drawings that begin each chapter are the work of Victor Kalin.

Copyright © 1978 by Litton Educational Publishing, Inc.
Library of Congress Catalog Card Number 77-12505
ISBN 0-442-20787-5

Printed in the United States of America

Published in 1978 by Van Nostrand Reinhold Company
A division of Litton Educational Publishing, Inc.
135 West 50th Street, New York, NY 10020, U.S.A.

Van Nostrand Reinhold Limited
1410 Birchmount Road, Scarborough, Ontario M1P 2E7, Canada

Van Nostrand Reinhold Australia Pty. Limited
17 Queen Street, Mitcham, Victoria 3132, Australia

Van Nostrand Reinhold Company Limited
Molly Millars Lane, Wokingham, Berkshire, England

1   3   5   7   9   11   13   15   16   14   12   10   8   6   4   2

Library of Congress Cataloging in Publication Data

Birren, Faber, 1900-
  Color and human response.

  Bibliography: p.
  Includes index.
  1. Color—Physiological effect.   2. Color vision.
3. Color—Psychological aspects.   4. Visual perception.
I. Title.
QP483.B57   155.9′11′45   77-12505
ISBN 0-442-20787-5

Contents

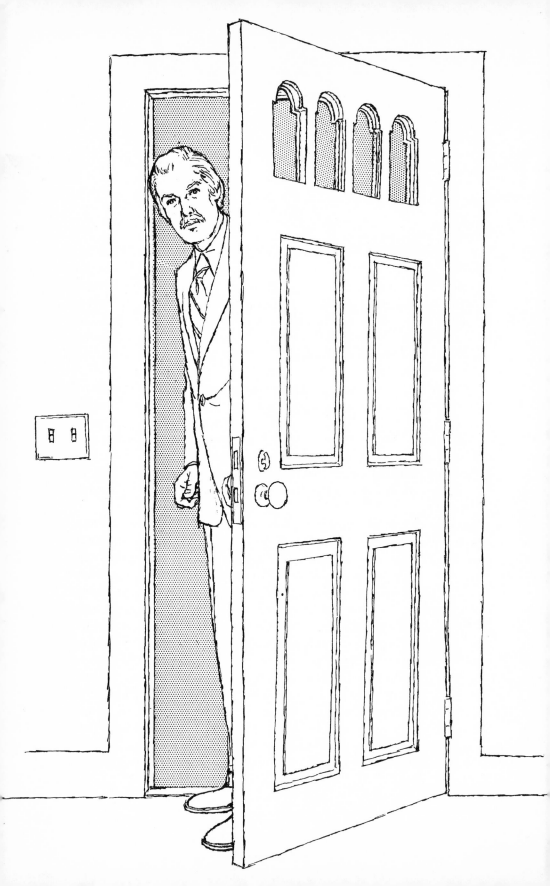

Preface

This is an informative book, and I have tried my best to make it readable. I believe it contains more material on its topic than has before been assembled in a single volume. It includes notes taken by me over a period of some thirty years. This effort has been inspired not in an attempt to be scholarly or erudite but simply because color and human response have always held a fascinating attraction for me. I wanted to know all I could, and I was eager to apply all possible knowledge to my professional work as a color consultant.

After an early training in art I began to study people in their numerous and diverse reactions to color. This meant less physics and chemistry than history, tradition, mythology, mysticism, symbolism, psychology, and aesthetics. Most of my books (25 in all) have been directed toward the human side of color, toward its ancient and modern biological and cultural influence, toward practical applications in modern life, and toward new modes of color expression founded on recent inquiries into perception.

This has caused me some grief, for, as a writer on the subject of color, I have been difficult to classify—and easy to criticize. In a book like this one, for example, a mystic might say that I have been too skeptical, and a rationalist might acuse me of being too mystical. I am not bothered. Frankly, my aim in virtually all I have written on color has had one direct focus—people. If people in some attitudes hold esoteric views and if others demand only what can be fully substantiated, they are in both cases human beings. I love them all and am quite willing to hear them out, whether I agree with them or not.

Committees to investigate the physiological, visual, and psychological influences of color have been set up by such organizations as the Illuminating Engineering Society and the Inter-Society Color Council, the latter group composed of representatives from 28 different fields. Conferences are being held in the United States and Canada, and in 1976 an international congress on Color Dynamics took place in Budapest, Hungary. A first annual meeting of the American Society for Photobiology, which has much to do with light and color, occurred in Sarasota, Florida in 1973.

Such groups have a strong, *personal* concern with the effects of light and color. Biologically considered, such effects are finding therapeutic applications to a number of major and minor human ills and are serving as visual aids in diagnosis. Psychologically considered, color in particular is needed in contrived environments to counteract sensory deprivation, which can lead to no end of physiological and psychological disturbances. Legions of persons are being "cooped up" in large housing developments, convalescent homes, and homes for the aged. Mortals troubled by the tensions and crises of the times are packing mental institutions. Even among normal human beings engaged in normal occupations megastructures are being built and planned, underground and undersea communities that may keep masses of people out of nature and away from sunlight. And dedicated creatures may be confined in giant space capsules for days, weeks, and even months and years. Science may be able to keep them in good shape physically, but what will keep them from going mad mentally?

For all these directions it is my hope that this book will offer some advice on the benefits of color and at the same time serve as a convenient reference to the numerous sources of information that I have encountered in the course of my studies.

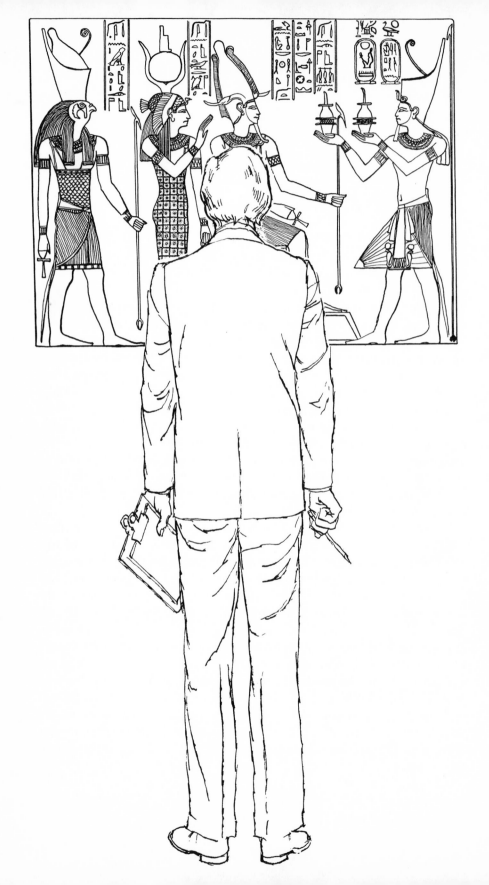

I. The Historical Background

In these days of world travel people in all walks of life—business, professional, scientific, and just average tourists—are being treated to the art of ancient times from cave drawings to the archaeological remains of Egypt, Chaldea, India, China, Greece, Central America. What a wonderful sense of color had early man! The assumption, an erroneous one, is that early man somehow needed beauty in his life and was inspired to surround himself with charming color in all art forms—architecture, painting, decoration, sculpture, textiles, ceramics. While the ancient may well have had a devout sense of color, his attitude toward the spectrum was far from aesthetic alone, as this chapter will attempt to explain.

Virtually up to the Renaissance man had symbolism, mystery, and magic in mind. What he did with color was dictated to him by mystics, philosophers, priests. By no means did he give free fancy to his imagination. Cosmetics gave distinction to race. Jewelry consisted of purposeful amulets. Tomb and temple decorations told stories. Even abstract decoration had meaning associated with gods, life and death, rain, harvest, victory in war.

What is obvious and remarkable is that the palette used by ancient man was simple, and direct and that it hardly differed in choice of hue anywhere in the ancient world: red, gold, yellow, green, blue, purple, white, and black. Egyptian paintboxes, to be found in museums, had sections for about eight colors, seldom more. As to Greek color, the reader may be surprised by this quotation from eminent British portraitist Sir William Beechey (1753–1839) regarding Greek polychrome decoration: "We observe that the practice we allude to [the use of similar colors on similar elements in decoration and sculpture] does not appear . . . to be the result of any occasional caprice or fancy, but of a generally established system; for the colors of the several parts do not seem to have materially varied in any two instances with which we are acquainted. . . . We can scarcely doubt that one particular color was appropriated by general consent or practice to each of the several parts of the buildings."

1

COLOR AND MAN HIMSELF

I do not exaggerate when I say that ancient man surrounded himself with color and in turn was surrounded by it. All civilizations since the beginning of man's existence worshipped the sun, and from the sun came light and color. In the Hindu *Upanishads,* which date back to centuries before Christ, man was described thus: "There are in his body the veins called Hita, which are as small as a hair divided a thousandfold, full of white, blue, yellow, green, and red." And again, "Symmetry of form, beauty of color, strength and compactness of the diamond, constitute bodily perfection." The father of Svetaketu counseled, not without a sense of humor: "Man is like a pillow-case. The color of one may be red, that of another blue, that of a third black, but all contain the same cotton. So it is with man—one is beautiful, another is black, a third holy, a fourth wicked, but the divine One dwells within them all." (Many of the quotations from the Hindu *Upanishads* and other ancient oriental religions are drawn from the excellent book *The Bible of the World* by Friedrich Spiegelberg.)

In his *Descent of Man* Darwin wrote, "We know . . . that the color of skin is regarded by the men of all races as a highly important element in their beauty." Perhaps for obvious reasons the Egyptians considered themselves members of the red race, used red cosmetics, and exaggerated the color red in depictions of themselves. Yellow was for the Asiatics, white for the peoples of the north, and black for the Negro.

In Sir Richard Burton's *Arabian Nights* is found the "Tale of the Ensorcelled Prince," in which the wife of the Prince cast a spell upon the inhabitants of the Black Islands: "And the citizens, who were of four different faiths, Moslems, Nazarene, Jew and Magian, she transformed by her enchantments into fishes; the Moslems are the white, the Magians the red, the Christians blue, and the Jews yellow."

THE ELEMENTS OF THE WORLD

Primitive man's idea of the universe was conceived in terms of elements, and this has persisted into modern times. I quote again from the Hindu *Upanishads* these amusing references to the significance of red, white, and black: "Of all living things there are indeed three origins only, that which springs from an egg, that which springs from a living being, and that which springs from a germ. . . .

"The red color of burning fire is the color of fire, the white color of fire is the color of water, the black color of fire the color of earth. Thus vanishes what we call fire, as a mere variety, being a name, arising from speech. What is true is the three colors. The red color of the sun is the color of fire, the white of water, the black of earth. Thus vanishes what we call the sun, as a mere variety, being a name, arising from speech. What is true is the three colors. The red color of the moon is the color of fire, the white of water, the black of earth. Thus vanishes what we call the moon as a mere variety, being a name, arising from speech. What is true is the three colors. The red color of the lightning is the color of fire, the white of water, the black of earth. Thus vanishes what we call the lightning, as a mere variety, being a name, arising from speech. What is true is the three colors. . . .

"Great householders and great theologians of olden times who knew this have declared the same, saying, 'No one can henceforth mention to us anything which we have not heard, perceived, or known.' Out of these they knew all. Whatever they thought looked red, they knew was the color of fire. Whatever they thought looked white, they knew was the color of water. Whatever they thought looked black, they knew was the color of earth. Whatever they thought was altogether unknown, they knew was some combination of those three beings."

To the early Greeks there were four elements, still acknowledged by the mystics today and recognized by Leonardo da Vinci during the Renaissance. These were earth, fire, water, and air. Aristotle stated in *De Coloribus* (which may have been written by his disciple Theophrastus): "Simple colors are the proper colors of the elements, i.e. of fire, air, water, and earth. Air and water when pure are by nature white, fire (and the sun) yellow, and the earth is naturally white. The variety of hues which earth assumes is due to coloration by tincture, as is shown by the fact that ashes turn white when the moisture that tinged them is burnt out. It is true that they do not turn a pure white, but that is because they are tinged afresh, in the process of combustion, by smoke, which is black. . . . Black is the proper color of elements in process of transmutation. The remaining colors, it may easily be seen, arise from blending by mixture of these primary colors."

This viewpoint was accepted for many centuries. The Chinese, however, recognized five elements: earth, which was yellow; fire, red; water, black; wood, green; and metal, white, the element air being omitted. C. A. S. Williams in his *Outlines of Chinese Symbolism* remarks, "Upon these five elements or perpetually active principles of Nature the whole scheme of Chinese philosophy . . . is based."

The Jewish historian Josephus in the first century A.D. associated white with earth, red with fire, purple with water, and yellow with air. Then the great Leonardo da Vinci *fifteen centuries* later declared in his *A Treatise on Painting*: "The first of all simple colors is white, though philosophers will not acknowledge either white or black to be colors; because the first is the cause, or the receiver, of colors, the other totally deprived of them. But as painters cannot do without either, we shall place them among the others; and according to this order of things, white will be the first, yellow the second, green the third, blue the fourth, red the fifth, and black the sixth. We shall set down white for the representative of light, without which no color can be seen; yellow for the earth; green for water; blue for air; red for fire; and black for total darkness."

THE QUARTERS OF THE WORLD

In human response to color it is curious to note man's concept of the earth as having four quarters or directions, each of which has a symbolic color. Here again, this had nothing essentially to do with beauty but with magic and symbolic meaning. The Egyptian pharaoh wore a white crown as a token of his dominion over upper Egypt and a red crown for lower Egypt.

Among the peoples of Tibet the world was conceived as a high mountain. This the Mongols called Sumur. From the beginning of time the earth grew. Its summit rose to a height beyond the reach of man and hence provided a convenient dwelling place for the gods. An old legend relates: "In the beginning was only water and a frog, which gazed into the water. God turned this animal over and created the world on its belly. On each foot he built a continent, but on the navel of the frog he founded the Sumur Mountain. On the summit of this mountain is the North Star."

The Tibetan world mountain was shaped like a pyramid with its top broken off. The sides facing the four points of the compass were hued and shone like jewels. To the north was yellow, to the south blue, to the east white, to the west red. In each of these directions was a continent within a salty sea. The continents and the isles that stood about them had shapes that resembled the faces of the people who dwelt upon them. The people to the south, India, China, Mongolia, had oval faces. Those to the north had square faces. Those to the west had rounded faces. The faces of those to the east were crescent-shaped.

Equally intriguing was the Chinese vision of Four Heavenly Kings. Mo-li Shou, the guardian of the north, had a black face. Within his bag was a creature that assumed the form of a snake or white winged elephant and devoured men. Mo-li Hung, the guardian of the south, had a red face. He held the umbrella of chaos, at the elevation of which there was universal darkness, thunder, and earthquakes. Mo-li Ch'ing, the guardian of the east, had a green face. His expression was ferocious and his beard like copper wire. With his magic sword, the Blue Cloud, he caused a black wind that produced tens of thousands of spears to pierce and destroy the bodies of men. Mo-li Hai, the guardian of the west, had a white face. At the sound of his guitar all the world listened, and the camps of his enemies caught fire.

The quarters of the earth no doubt referred to the movement of the sun from morning to noon to evening, with the fourth direction being that region of the universe that the sun did not trespass. From Egypt to Tibet to China and thence around the world symbolism for the points of the compass was repeated. The Irish of old appointed black to the north, white to the south, purple to the east, dun color to the west. The Mayans of Yucatan chose white for the north, yellow for the south, red for the east, and black for the west. Among American Indians (Apache, Cherokee, Chippewa, Creek, Zuñi) colors were assigned to the four directions, and these designations might be different from tribe to tribe.

Thousands of years ago, according to one fable, the Navahos dwelt in a land surrounded by high mountains. The rise and fall of these mountains created day and night. The eastern mountains were white and caused the day. The western mountains were yellow and brought twilight. The northern mountains were black and covered the earth in darkness, while the blue mountains to the south created dawn.

The American Indian also had color designations for a lower world, which was generally black, and an upper world, which had many colors. All this symbolism was a part of his art. The tattooing on his face and the colors on his masks, effigies, huts were full of meaning and not mere products of an artistic temperament. He applied these hues of the compass to his songs, ceremonies, prayers, and games. Even today the Hopi in executing a dry painting is a mystic before he is an artist. Religiously he first places his yellow color, which represents the north. Then, in order, he places the green or blue of the west, the red of the south, and lastly the white of the east.

What many today may look upon as charming and romantic in the culture of the American Indian probably had its origin in mysticism and symbolism. He was not merely "enthralled" by the beauty of color but attributed definite magic to it. To the Indian red symbolized day and black symbolized night—always. Red, yellow, and black were masculine colors; white, blue, and green were feminine. Certain tribes related hues to the four Indian elements, fire, wind, water, and earth. To the Cherokee red signified success and triumph. Blue denoted tribulation and defeat. White stood for peace and happiness, black for death. Prayer sticks were bright with green to call the rain and livid with red before the war.

THE GODS

All religions, primitive or otherwise, have looked upon their gods in terms of luminous color, for the gods invariably dwelt in heaven from whence shone the sun, moon, stars, and rainbow. (Earth gods were usually mortal or evil.) God was often the sun itself. Let me offer a few brief examples, taken mostly from my book *The Story of Color.*

In Egypt the sun itself was Ra and Osiris. (Isis was the moon.) Its symbol might be gold, yellow, or red. In parts of India the color was said to be blue. The name SOL-OM-ON is said to be the name of the sun in three languages.

In ancient Greece yellow or gold was assigned to Athena. Her temple was the Parthenon at Athens. Red was sacred to Ceres, goddess of the harvest. Dionysus, the wine god, had a red face. Iris was the rainbow.

In India the color of Buddha was yellow or gold. According to Buddhist scriptures, "No sooner has he set his right foot within the city-gate than the rays of six different colors which issue from his body rose hither and thither over palaces and pagodas, and decked them, as it were, with the yellow sheen of gold, or with the colors of a painting." Yet if Buddha pondered over the sins of men, he might wear red. "And the Blessed one, putting on a tunic of double red cloth, and binding on his girdle, and throwing his upper robe over his right shoulder, would go thither and sit down, and for a while remain solitary, and plunged in meditation."

In the Bible, the Old and New Testament, there are many color references. Colors are described in relation to the Tabernacle in the Wilderness, which was to have linen curtains in blue, purple, and scarlet. The Lord commanded Moses to "Speak unto the children of Israel, that they bring me an offering: of every man that giveth it willingly with his heart ye shall take my offering. And this is the offering ye shall take of them: gold, and silver, and brass. And blue, and purple, and scarlet, and fine linen, and goats' hair, and rams' skins dyed red, and badgers' skins, and shittim wood, oil for the light, spices for anointing oil, and for sweet incense, onyx stones, and stones to be set in the ephod, and in the breastplate."

God the Father's color was blue, according to Exodus. "Then up went Moses, and Aaron, and Nadab, and Abihu, and seventy of the elders of Israel; and they saw the God of Israel: and there was under his feet as it were a paved work of sapphire stone, and as it were the very heaven for clearness." Legend tells that the Ten Commandments were inscribed on blue sapphire, and a red carbuncle was at the prow of Noah's ark.

Ezekiel likens God unto a rainbow: "As the appearance of the bow that is in the cloud in the day of rain, so was the appearance of the brightness round about. This was the appearance of the likeness of the glory of the Lord." And Ezekiel continues, "And above the firmament that was over their heads was the likeness of a throne, as the appearance of a sapphire stone: and upon the likeness of the throne was the likeness as the appearance of a man above it. And I saw as the color of amber."

Green emerald is associated with Christ. According to St. John the Divine, "And he that sat was to look upon like a jasper and a sardine throne: and there was a rainbow round about the throne, in sight like unto an emerald." Blue among Christians is most often associated with the Virgin Mary.

Jewish and Christian color symbolism still exists in the rites of these religions. As vestments in different colors are changed from season to season, the colors may delight the eye, but they tell of feasts and passions that were meaningful before they were beautiful.

PLANETS AND STARS

The ancient had a vital interest in the universe, the sun, stars, and planets, for to him they regulated all life. Most surviving archaeological structures from centuries past consisted of temples and shrines, not homes. Important monuments needed to be elegant and dedicated to divine powers, not common man. One truly remarkable finding is the close and mystical relationship between color and architecture. Egyptian buildings frequently had green floors like the meadows of the Nile and blue ceilings like the sky.

Let me refer to two splendid examples of color symbolism in ancient temples. Many years ago Dr. C. Leonard Woolley, on the joint expedition of the British Museum and the Museum of Pennsylvania, unearthed the ancient *ziggurat,* the Mountain of God, at Ur between Bagdad and the Persian Gulf, one of the oldest buildings in the world. Dating back to 2300 B.C., it was thought to be the original home of Abraham, founded before the Flood. The tower measured 200 feet in length, 150 feet in width, and was originally about 70 feet high. It was built in four stages, a great, solid mass of brickwork. Woolley found an absence of straight lines. Horizontal planes bulged outward; vertical planes were slightly convex—a subtlety once thought to be of Greek origin and quite evident in the Parthenon. The lowest stage of the tower was black, the uppermost red. The shrine was covered with blue glazed tile, the roof with gilded metal. Woolley writes, "These colors had mystical significance and stood for the various divisions of the universe, the dark underworld, the habitable earth, the heavens and the sun."

More pretentious *ziggurats* have been unearthed. In the fifth century B.C. Herodotus wrote of Ecbatana: "The Medes built the city now called Ecbatana, the walls of which are of great size and strength, rising in circles one within the other. The plan of the place is, that each of the walls should out-top the one beyond it by the battlements. The nature of the ground, which is a gentle hill, favors this arrangements in some degree, but it is mainly effected by art. The number of the circles is seven, the royal palace and the treasuries standing within the last. The circuit of the outer wall is very nearly the same with that of Athens. On this wall the battlements are white, of the next black, of the third scarlet, of the fourth blue, of the fifth orange; all these are colored with paint. The last two have their battlements coated respectively with silver and gold. All these fortifications Deïoces had caused to be raised for himself and his own palace."

Herodotus, to all indications, referred to the great temple of Nebuchadnezzar at Barsippa, the Birs Nimroud. Uncovered in modern times, its bricks bear the stamp of the Babylonian monarch who apparently rebuilt it in the seventh century B.C. It was 272 feet square at its base and rose in seven stages, each stage being set back from a central point. Of this building James Fergusson writes: "This temple, as we know from the decipherment of the cylinders which were found on its angles, was dedicated to the seven planets or heavenly spheres, and we find it consequently adorned with the colors of each. The lower, which was also richly panelled, was black, the color of Saturn; the next, orange, the color of Jupiter; the third, red, emblematic of Mars; the fourth yellow, belonging to the Sun; the fifth and sixth, green and blue respectively, as dedicated to Venus and Mercury, and the upper probably white, that being the color belonging to the Moon, whose place in the Chaldean system would be uppermost."

This use of color, of course, is quite remote in spirit and intent from the modern choice of color for buildings. I think it bears repeating that the ancient was a mystic before he was an artist. There is clear evidence that he did little to express his own personal feelings but instead carried out the complex directions of others. The face of the Sphinx was colored red. Also so colored were the ziggurats of Asia Minor and all early Greek architecture and sculpture—and the Inca, Mayan, and Toltec pyramids, temples, and shrines of Mexico and Central and South America.

CULTURE

The story of the early history of color could go on and on. Other of my books may be consulted by the interested reader. To end this chapter, here are some miscellaneous notes on color and culture that continue to tell of the symbolic and practical role of color in human life of the past. (Further historical reviews will be encountered in the introductions of chapters that follow.)

One may recall references to the Golden Age, Imperial Purple, the Mauve Decade. In China the royal color of the Sung Dynasty (960–1127 A.D.) was brown, the Ming Dynasty (1368–1644) green, the Ch'ing Dynasty (1644–1911) yellow. In Rome the emperor wore purple to personify Jupiter, and the color was exclusively his.

In India there were originally four castes: the Brahmans, the Kshatriyas, the Vaisyas, and the Sudras. As the story goes, mankind once comprised four races. From the mouth of the creator came the Brahmans. From his arms came the Kshatriyas. From his thighs came the Vaisyas. And from his feet came the Sudras. These were the four *varnas*, a word which means "color" in the Sanskrit language.

The Brahmans were white. They were supposed to study, to teach, to sacrifice for themselves, and to be priests to others. They gave alms and received alms. They were privileged and of the sacred class. The Kshatriyas were red. They were meant to study but not to teach, to sacrifice for themselves but not to officiate as priests. They were to give but not to receive alms. Their class was militant, and they governed and fought the wars. The Vaisyas were yellow. They were of the mercantile class. They were to study, sacrifice for themselves, give alms, cultivate the fields, breed cattle, trade, and lend money at interest. The Sudras were black. They were of the servile class and were to obtain their livelihood by laboring for others. They might practice the useful arts, but they were not to study the holy Vedas.

Colors were assigned to the planets and the signs of the Zodiac, and they still are by modern astrologers. (Recall the description of Ecbatana by Herodotus previously quoted.)

There were colors for heraldry, flags, and emblems, traditions and symbolism that survive to this day, as in religious vestments and the trappings of education in major faculties: scarlet for theology, blue for philosophy, white for arts and letters, green for medicine, purple for law, golden yellow for science, orange for engineering, pink for music.

Among primitive tribes even today there are color rituals having to do with birth and death, circumcision in boys, puberty in girls, protection for the lion slayer and man slayer. Bodies are painted, amulets worn, magic colors displayed in ceremonial dress. There was wonder in ancient color—and beauty by coincidence.

Following are a few interesting references to the mythological and symbolic importance of color in the lives of people through the ages. From birth to death color charmed the life of the primitive and the ancient. The purple baptismal stole of the Christian priest in Europe, the Creek Indian boy smeared with white clay at his circumcision—in all lands and nations color was one of man's first blessings and the last sacred benison to shroud his cadaver. As he grew into childhood, his body was protected by talismans, his home rid of evil through the magic of hue. Almost everything that related to his civilization and culture was associated with the colors of the rainbow.

Life was precious, blood and death tragic and awesome. Man's struggle was endless against the forces of nature, the will of the gods, the curse of demons. He was born from the body of a women, and when he died his flesh rotted and turned black. He was circumspect. The blood of puberty frightened him. He secluded his daughter. She must be covered with red pigment, buried in the ground, or immured in a hut. She must come forth with her face painted red and white lest she give birth to monsters after her marriage. She must marry, and the ceremony must be the most jubilant of rites. It must be colorful, and the bride and groom must be preserved by the magic power of hue throughout their marital years.

Among the ancient Jews the marriage ceremony was performed under the Talis, a golden silk robe supported by four pillars. Around this the bride walked seven times in memory of the siege of Jericho. In India red paint and even blood were used. Six days before her wedding the Hindu bride wore old, tattered yellow garments to drive away evil spirits. Her clothing at the ceremony was yellow, and so too were the robes of the priest. And, once married, the wife wore yellow upon the return of her husband from a long journey.

In China the bride wore red embroidered with dragons. She was carried in a red marriage chair adorned with lanterns inscribed with the groom's family name in red. She held a red parasol. Red firecrackers were exploded on her behalf. During the rite bride and bridegroom drank a pledge of wine and honey from two cups, which were tied together by a red cord.

In Japan the daughter of a man who fed a thousand white hares in his house would marry a prince. In the Dutch East Indies red or yellow rice was sprinkled over the bridegroom to keep his soul from flying away. Red was also the color of a love potion, and, if the names of boy and girl were written on white paper with the blood of a red hen, the girl would become infatuated when touched by it.

Red and yellow—these were the marriage hues of Egypt, the Orient, Russia, the Balkans—and they still are. In the western countries blue was and is worshipful. An old English rhyme, familiar to everyone, cautions the bride to wear

Something old and something new.

Something borrowed and something blue.

If the ordinance of marriage was jubilant, the ritualism of death was ponderous, elaborate, and august. Man faced the greatest of all mysteries and ventured into domains from which no one had ever returned. Though an impeccable mortal life might assure his salvation, even the sinful might not die forever. Yet, good or evil, the dead must be buried. His family must prepare his shroud and equip his tomb with the necessary accouterments for his expedition to the realm of the immortals.

In wilder countries the native was superstitious about the treachery of demons. When a Nandi of eastern Africa killed the member of another tribe, he painted one side of his body, spear, and sword red and the other side white. This protected him from the ghost of his victim. In Fiji a native who clubbed another man to death was smeared with red from head to foot by the chief of his tribe. In South Africa the lion killer painted his body white, went into seclusion for four days, and then returned to the village with his flesh coated red.

Black, however, is the universal color of mourning among nearly all western peoples, for it has the very appearance of death. Certain primitives dye their teeth black after the passing of a relative. In England the garments of widows are white faced with black. Servants in mourning for their masters wear black, unrelieved by any other color, even to the buttons.

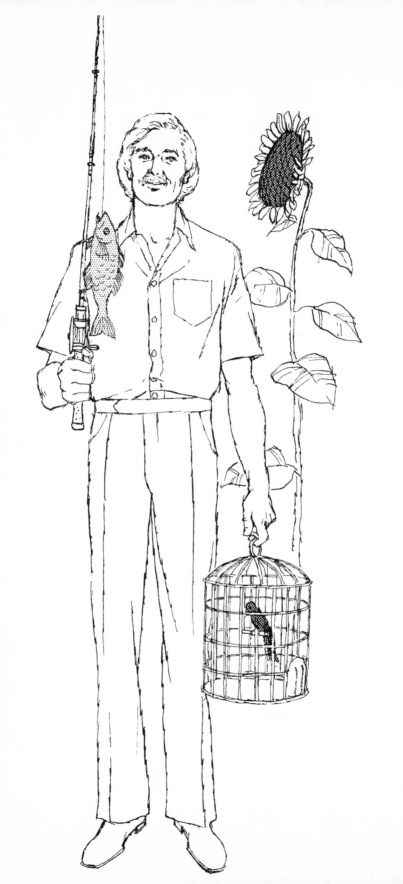

II. Biological Response

This chapter is concerned with manifestations of white and colored light as they affect living things. Richard J. Wurtman states, "It seems clear that light is the most important environmental input, after food, in controlling bodily function." Let me lead into the biological implications of light by commenting first on other forms of electromagnetic energy. If the following few paragraphs seem academic to a sophisticated reader, please forgive.

The full extent of electromagnetic energy, including visible light and color, is vast. All this energy travels at a speed of about 186,000 miles a second, as measured by Albert Michelson several decades ago. While speed is the same, wavelengths of the energy differ as measured from crest to crest. Though measurements of these waves involve thousands of feet at one end of the electromagnetic spectrum to infinitesimal fractions of an inch at the other, the scientific world is quite satisfied that its figures are accurate.

BELOW VISIBLE LIGHT

Long waves are used for wireless, as developed by Guglielmo Marconi back at the turn of the century. They are used for long-distance communication. Marconi first transmitted signals across the Atlantic in 1901. This marked the beginning of a vast world of "wireless" communication that today serves indispensable purposes in modern life. Marconi received the Nobel Prize in 1909. Next longest are induction heat waves, which can be used to raise temperatures in order to harden metals.

Commercial (AM) broadcasting waves come next. They have the ability to bounce back from the ionosphere of the sky and thus to travel around the earth. Shortwave bands are used for general broadcasting, police cars, taxicabs, and the recent citizen-band (CB) radios. Waves used in diathermy, which can generate heat through electrodes clamped to the body to relieve arthritis, neuralgia, are shorter still.

FM radio, television, radar are transmitted as the waves grow shorter. Because this energy penetrates the ionosphere, it is not thrown back. By launching satellites above the earth, however, these stations in the sky can be used to reflect waves back like mirrors. Microwave towers, seen everywhere across the land, are used to transmit messages from point to point in straight lines.

Infrared waves will penetrate heavy atmosphere. Cameras sensitive to this energy can take pictures of a world that is otherwise invisible to human eyes. They can also be focused like a rifle to pick out anything emitting heat, such as the bodies of enemy soldiers (or bucolic cows). Radiant heat from radiators and infrared lamps has waves far below visible light.

ABOVE VISIBLE LIGHT

The visible region of the electromagnetic spectrum runs the gamut from red through orange, yellow, green, blue, and violet. It fades out at longwave ultraviolet. Rays of coherent visible light (often red) have been concentrated in the laser beam and used to strike the moon, establish channels of communication, cut metal, drill holes in diamonds, and repair detached retinas in the human eye—among a constantly increasing list of wonders. Laser beams are also a part of modern holography, which creates three-dimensional images without the use of conventional methods of photography.

Long ultraviolet waves produce fluorescence in many substances and are used for the modern fluorescent lamp. Shorter ultraviolet waves tan the skin (and cause cancer with too much exposure) and help to produce vitamin D. Still shorter UV radiation will kill germs and sterilize material substances, water, and air.

Grenz rays, or "soft" x rays, are used therapeutically for some skin diseases. Shorter x rays are used for diagnostic purposes, and still "harder" x rays to treat deep-seated tumors and cancers within the body. The gamma rays discovered by Pierre and Marie Curie in 1898 are used to treat much lethal cancer. The emanations of nuclear fission, associated with the atom bomb, bombardment of the atom nucleus, and the nuclear powerplant, are shorter still. The shortest of all waves, the cosmic rays that pervade the universe, are something of a mystery.

THE HAZARDS OF ELECTROMAGNETIC ENERGY

If all waves of electromagnetic energy were visible to the human eye, they would surely have the aspect of a blinding snowstorm driving at a person from all directions. What hazards are involved? Man is very much aware of the dangers of undue exposure to nuclear energy, radium and x rays, and excessive ultraviolet. Nuclear powerplants are constantly under public attack, and accidents here could indeed have disastrous results. But what about energy that is presumably harmless? Color-TV sets emit unwanted radiation and today are legally required to be adequately provided with shields. Such energy can be felt if the hand is held close to the screen. Microwave ovens have also been under surveillance and must be shielded. As one suspicious electronics engineer cautioned, "The best way is to prepare the food, put it in the oven, close the door, turn it on, and hurry out of the room!"

People are commonly exposed to radiation from TV sets; AM and FM radio; telephone relay towers; police, weather, and airport radio and radar systems; citizen-band radios, electric motors and generators, high-power transmission lines—not to mention the better-known hazards. John Ott, in this book *Health and Light,* writes, "There have also been reports from Manitoba, Canada, of dairy herds, located within two miles of telephone microwave relay towers, giving considerably less milk, poultry producing only a fraction of their usual egg quota and flocks of chickens going into sudden, unexplained hysterical stampedes."

In the news today are articles on dangers surrounding the exhaustion of oxygen in the ozone layer above the earth's atmosphere, which is an effective absorber of lethal ultraviolet radiation. This oxygen is said to be consumed by supersonic airplanes, gas from aerosol sprays, atom-bomb tests. If excessive ultraviolet were to reach the earth, much plant and animal life would be destroyed, and man would need adequate protection. Less ominous is concern over the biological effects of artificial-light sources (which will be further discussed in the next chapter). There is talk of "light pollution" where balanced, or "full-spectrum," light does not exist. A person has good reason to be suspicious of illumination that does not measure up to that of nature in sunlight and skylight. This point will be emphasized in the following pages. I shall discuss the importance of color to plants, insects, fish, birds, animals, and human beings.

PLANTS

Considerable research has been conducted on the effects of color on plant life. Among the prominent investigators in the field have been H. A. Borthwick of the U.S. Department of Agriculture, Stuart Dunn of the University of New Hampshire, and R. van der Veen and G. Meijer of the Philips Research Laboratories in Holland. Borthwick noted an antagonism between visible red light and invisible infrared. Red would cause lettuce seed to sprout, for example, while infrared would put the sprouts back to sleep. Similarly, red would inhibit the flowering of the short-day plants and promote that of long-day ones. Van der Veen and Meijer reported that there was maximum absorption of red light and hence maximum plant action. Blue had similar effects, but yellow and green were neutral or reduced activity, and short ultraviolet would destroy the plant.

What is unusual is that plants seem most receptive to red and blue and are inactive to yellow and yellow-green. The human eye, however, finds maximum sensitivity (visibility) to yellow and yellow-green. In a greenhouse under artificial light weak green illumination is "safe" for plants, for there is little if any plant response to it. This light is to the plant physiologist "what the ruby light was for the photographer," according to Van der Veen and Meijer.

In correspondence with the author, Stuart Dunn of the plant-physiology laboratory at the University of New Hampshire has discussed the growth of tomato seedlings: "The yield by the warm white lamps was highest of all the commercially available fluorescent lamps. Next to it stood that of the blue and pink lamps. Green and red were low. The experimental 'high intensity' of red lamps produced the highest yield of all. Stem growth (elongation) is promoted especially by the yellow part of the spectrum. . . ." but "Succulence is increased by the long wavelengths (red) and decreased by blue light."

Chrysanthemum flowers can be made to bloom early by covering the plants with cloth for part of the day to reduce the length of their exposure to light. The colorful leaves of poinsettias can be similarly controlled by adding hours of light at certain times. To quote from an article by Victor A. Greulach: "Among the common short-day plants are asters, ragweeds, dahlias, cosmos, poinsettia, chrysanthemum, cypress vine, nasturtiums, soy beans, tobacco, and all the early spring flowers such as violets and bloodroots. Most garden vegetables and farm crops are long-day plants.

Wheat grows rapidly under long days. By using electric light to increase the day-length three generations of wheat have been grown in one year. The extremely long summer days in Alaska are largely responsible for the large crops of hay, wheat, potatoes, and vegetables grown there. It is principally due to the longer days in the northern part of the central valley of California that oranges from that district are ripe and ready for the market several weeks earlier than those grown four hundred miles farther south.

"We usually think of everblooming or everbearing plants as being particular species of varieties, as of roses or strawberries, but many plants may be made into everbloomers by keeping the length-of-day within their natural flowering range. For most plants this range is quite narrow, so we have few everblooming plants in the temperate latitudes, where the day-lengths are constantly changing. In the tropics, where the day-lengths are at or near twelve hours all year, everbloomers are the rule rather than the exception, just as you would expect."

If natural cycles of night and day are not adjusted to the needs of a plant, trouble may be encountered. John Ott reports on the poinsettia: "I heard a story from Honolulu that the Chamber of Commerce there had run into . . . difficulty when an attempt was made to turn floodlights on some of the poinsettias in one of the parks. It is also known that a street-light, too near a greenhouse of poinsettias, will cause them all kinds of blooming problems."

Street lamps near a tree have been known to cause untimely death, perhaps by urging the tree to undergo growth that is unnatural to it. Ott has further curiosities to report about plants and light: "It is interesting to place a night-blooming cereus and a day-blooming cactus side by side in a totally dark closet and note the blooms of the nocturnal plant open in the nighttime and then close during the daytime, while the diurnal plant responds oppositely, regardless of whether an ordinary incandescent light is on or off. Another good example is the way a sensitive-plant folds its leaves and lowers its branches at night and then resumes its daytime position as the sun rises the next morning. If the sensitive plant is placed in a dark closet during the daytime, the leaves remain open in daytime position until the sun sets outdoors. They will resume their daytime position when the sun rises even though they remain in the dark closet." One wonders what magic accounts for these phenomena.

In France irradiation of potato plants with red light has stimulated germination, and satisfactory crop yields have been achieved. Growing flowering plants completely under artificial light is fast becoming a national hobby in the United States, making the mystery and magic of color more impressive to the layman.

INSECTS

Many insects have a fair sense of color: they are insensitive to red but sensitive to yellow, green, blue, violet, and into ultraviolet, which is invisible to man. A group of researchers, H. B. Weiss, F. A. Soroci, and E. E. McCoy, Jr., tested about 4,500 insects, mostly beetles, and found that 72 percent reacted positively to some wavelength, 33 percent to yellow-green, 14 percent to violet-blue, 11 percent to blue, and 11 percent to ultraviolet. Few showed any attraction to warm colors. "It thus appears that in general the shorter wavelengths of light are more stimulating and attractive, whereas the longer wavelengths are considerably less stimulative and perhaps repellent in nature to coleopterous forms of life [beetles]."

Insects are able to see into the ultraviolet and beyond into frequencies approaching x rays. Von Frish found that bees could see the difference between a blue and a gray of the same brightness but were confused when the same test was performed with red. Not only does the insect have a different range of color vision than birds or man, but flowers may also have a different appearance to them. Some flowers (red portulaca) reflect ultraviolet, while others (red zinnia) do not. Further, the patterns on the wings of some butterflies and moths will have a different formation under natural daylight than under ultraviolet light.

Yellow electric light bulbs, advertised as insect repellents, in fact merely lack attraction, whereas ultraviolet is a decided lure. Mosquitoes seem to be repelled by light colors and attracted by deep colors. When boxes were lined with navy blue, pink, gray, and yellow flannel, the blue boxes harbored far more of the insects than the pink or yellow.

FISH

Gordon Lynn Walls in *The Vertebrate Eye* wrote, "No fish are known *not* to have color vision." He further concluded that "Fishes generally seem either to shun red or to prefer it decidedly." In water red radiation is quickly absorbed, whereas blue and ultraviolet are not.

John Ott of the Environmental Health and Light Research Institute has studied higher forms of marine life. He has observed the effects of different wavelengths and light intensities on tropical fish. Young produced under pinkish fluorescent light were 80 percent female and 20 percent male; no young were produced under bluish fluorescent light. Even feeble amounts of light will affect the normal development of fish. Ott discusses the death rate among brook-trout eggs at the New York State Hatchery, which suddenly rose to 90 percent from under 10 percent: "Dr. Alfred Perlmutter of New York University traced the cause to installation of new 40-watt fluorescent lights in the ceiling. Another investigator, working with rainbow trout, found that the violet and blue components of white or visible light are more deadly than green, yellow and orange bands."

BIRDS

Birds have excellent color vision, particularly of red. Bird migration is said to be influenced by length of day. As summer days grow shorter, something within the bird (possibly through the pituitary gland) urges it to fly to more favorable climates. This may happen even when fall crops are ripe with seed and insects are abundant.

Dutch and Japanese farmers expose songbirds to extra illumination in order to induce singing. An English scientist found starlings living in and around Picadilly Circus in London to be sexually active at a time when other starlings at Oxford were not. The light of the great white way was assumed to be the cause. To increase egg production in chickens and ducks, extra light is often used to supplement the duration of daylight.

A color repellent for birds? Poisoned grain spread in a field to kill rats (which are colorblind) was eaten indiscriminately by birds. If the poisoned seeds were dyed green, the rats would see no difference, but the birds would tend to disregard them as unripe. The British have considered the use of a purple colorant on airfields to discourage birds if not to drive them away.

ANIMALS

Length of day has similar effects on animals. According to Friedrich Ellinger, length of daylight seems to be the most important of all features in stimulating sexual activity—or inhibiting it. Ellinger reports the following in his *The Biological Fundamentals of Radiation Therapy*. Horses and donkeys reproduce during seasons of long daylight, with a decrease in sexual activity from October to January. When mares are exposed to additional illumination during the winter months, ovarian activity may be affected. Fertility decreases with cattle, sheep, and pigs during the summer months. Here sexual activity is usually confined to autumn and winter.

Ellinger tells further of W. J. Sweetman, a researcher in Alaska, who "obtained an improvement in wintertime fertility by illuminating the animals [cows] 14 hours a day, whereas at this time of year daylight lasted from six to eight hours." Another scientist, H. J. von Schumann, found "that the number of hours of sunshine is the most important factor for the forming of horns" in stags. He assumed that light was absorbed through the hide of the deer, causing the formation of vitamin D and stimulating horn growth. T. H. Bissonnette, a zoologist, was able to get weasels to turn white in summer rather than in winter by regulating exposure to daylight. He also succeeded in making goats provide milk at times of the year when they were not wont to do so—through light control.

As to the *color* of light, according to Ott, breeders of chinchillas will have a relatively high percentage of males if the animals are kept under ordinary (warm) incandescent light and a correspondingly higher ratio of females if they are kept under daylight (bluish) incandescent light. The use of blue daylight bulbs has now become commercial practice. Perhaps the eternal problem of sex preference in human babies may one day be solved through the medium of colored light!

Ott describes a case study in which mink were reared behind different-colored plastic windows. Ordinarily mink are quite vicious, particularly during the mating period. Those kept behind pink plastic became increasingly aggressive, while those behind blue plastic became more docile and could be handled like house pets. All females became pregnant after mating. To draw an empirical conclusion, man as well as mink seems to be excited by red radiation and pacified by blue.

HUMAN BEINGS

Dr. Thomas R. C. Sisson has written, "Light does not merely lend illumination to human existence but exerts a powerful physical force, affecting many compounds within the body, some metabolic processes, the life and generation of cells—even the rhythms of life. Light is ubiquitous, it can be manipulated, and it is not entirely benign." What comes as a surprise to many is that *visible* light penetrates further into animal and human muscle and tissue than was once thought. While infrared also penetrates, ultraviolet does not and only affects the skin superficially (though vitally). Sisson concludes, "Substantial amounts [of visible light] will pass through skin, subcutaneous tissue, muscle and even central organs if the intensity is strong enough." E. E. Brunt and associates caused light to penetrate the skulls of sheep, dogs, and rabbits. They demonstrated "that light does reach the temporal lobes and hypothalamus in a variety of mammalian species." The hypothalamus, incidentally, is the part of the brain—at its base—that is believed to contain vital autonomic nerve centers and fibers that control such functions as respiration, heart action, and digestion. If it is affected by light, the animal naturally responds in favorable or adverse ways depending on its needs. In an article for *Endrocrinology* (72: 962, 1963) W. F. Ganong and others reached the conclusion that "environmental light can penetrate the mammalian skull in sufficient amount to activate photoelectric cells imbedded in the brain tissue." This means that light is essential to a healthful and normal life and that nature has evolved ways in which it affects the body through the tissues of the skin, the eyes, and even the skull itself.

LIGHT AND DARK RHYTHMS

Granted that light is essential to human existence, so are rhythms of light and dark. Lightness and darkness cause different physiological actions in the body. Body temperature, for example, will change. The action of light may induce the secretion of hormones into the bloodstream. Persons who fly by plane from west to east may feel spells of nausea, physical distress, and mental disturbance. Space travel may demand light-dark cycles of artificial illumination for the human system to keep in good shape—not just light but regulated exposures to light.

If day and night rhythms are disturbed or unusually prolonged, odd results may follow. Here are two examples. Among Eskimo women menstruation may cease during the long artic night, and the libido of Eskimo men may also be dormant. Lack of light in effect leads to a natural form of human hibernation. This is by no means a racial characteristic unique to Eskimos. The same effects seem to occur to any person exposed to alternately long periods of sunlight and darkness. With the onset of the long arctic winter human sexual desire fails. It is revived again with the dawn of spring. Girls of tribes in North Greenland may marry at fourteen or fifteen, but menstruation may not occur until they reach nineteen or twenty. Eskimo children are generally born nine months after the advent of spring and the return of the arctic sun.

In an article by Francis Woidich, "The Resonant Brain," reference is made to a South American village where the birth rate dropped after electric lights were installed. While the natives may have found other uses for the extra hours of light beside procreation, Dr. Edmond Dewan nontheless wrote a fascinating article: "On the Possibility of a Perfect Rhythm Method of Birth Control by Periodic Light Stimulation." With extra artificial light turned on during certain days of the month, the chance of conception might be minimized. If the illuminants were blue rather than red (which is said to be a sexual stimulant), further birth control might be effected.

LIGHT DEPRIVATION

Lack of light also has odd results. The blind, of course, will react to light through their skin just like anyone else. Miners working for long periods of time in darkness or semidarkness may have eye troubles, such as an uncontrolled rolling of the eyeballs.

The medical profession speaks of spasmus nutans in infants—failure to thrive. In a series of reported cases by Dr. William B. Rothney it is apparent that light, any light at all, is highly significant even to the newborn. A number of infants were hospitalized for failure to respond to care at home. While all indicated "evidence of parental neglect . . . examination of the homes showed that each of these babies spent most, if not all, of his time in a darkened environment." Perhaps the mother watched TV or preferred to be isolated from life or the world. In any event, when babies were exposed to light and were given love and affection, normal health and growth were resumed.

PROLONGED LIGHT

Conversely, constant, uninterrupted light may also cause trouble. Dr. T. R. C. Sisson, professor of Pediatrics and Director of Neonatal Research at Temple University School of Medicine in Philadelphia, has experimented on "Effects of Uncycled Light on Biologic Rhythm of Plasma Human Growth Hormone." Because constant response to light is difficult to endure, even among adults with their eyes closed, such exposure makes adjustment impossible among infants. Sisson tried periods of different exposures. Infants normally develop an "ultradian" rhythm to light and dark. He concluded that constant lighting in a hospital nursery (which is convenient for nurses) "either prevents or obliterates the circadian rhythm of plasma human growth hormone shown to be present in newborn infants under dark/light cycling, and suggests the impropriety of constant light in nurseries."

EFFECTS OF COLOR

Effects of color—biological, visual, psychological—are discussed in other chapters of this book. Sisson writes, "Elegant studies of the effects of constant dark or light environment, and light of differing spectral distributions have shown effects on organ size, growth patterns, and sexual maturation in some animal species, possibly including man."

How are the effects of *color* specifically to be measured? Most of my own work with color and people (and it has been quite extensive) has concentrated more on psychological and emotional than on biological reactions. As mentioned briefly in Chapter VI, the polygraph (lie detector) can be employed to measure respiration, pulse, palmar conductance (skin response), and other physiological actions, while the electroencephalograph (EEG) can be used to measure brain waves. Different effects of color have been verified again and again, and anyone doubting this either confesses to prejudice or is isolated from the findings of the modern scientific laboratory.

To go back into recent history, Sidney L. Pressey wrote an article on "The Influences of Color Upon Mental and Motor Efficiency." At this time, over 50 years ago, the testimony of chromotherapists like Edwin D. Babbitt still held credence despite the denials of the recognized medical profession. One by one Pressey knocked down the assertions of others before him. "It would seem reasonable to conclude that if color *does* have any fundamental mental and motor efficiency, the connection must be of a very general and elementary nature; brightness may stimulate, or red irritate and distract, but more specific effects are hardly to be expected." Another researcher, Herman Vollmer, in his article "Studies in Biological Effect of Colored Light," declared that "Nowhere can we find a common biological denominator for the various experimental data." For example, Vollmer disputed certain findings that the growth rate of rats was greater under red light. This led to a classical bit of naive humor: "The superiority in weight of the red animals at the end of the experiment is partly explained by pregnancy of one of the animals."

A common and truly unforgivable error in most color research is that many of those who conduct it may fail to realize that color effects are always temporary. Exposure to color does not cause reactions of any substantial duration. If a person is exposed to strong areas of any hue (or to bright light), there is an immediate reaction that can easily be measured instrumentally. The reaction to color is not unlike the reaction to alcohol, tobacco, coffee—up for a short period and then down. In fact, if red is stimulating (which it is), after a length of time bodily responses may fall *below* normal. To the question as to whether or not red is an exciting color the answer is "yes-maybe-no," depending on the element of time. The "functional" use of color by this writer in many applications, such as in mental institutions (see Chapter VIII), is designed around the use of a *variety* of colors in order to keep human responses continually active and to avoid visual adaptation or emotional monotony.

A FEW CONCLUSIONS

In the main there are different biological reactions to the two extremes of the spectrum, red and green or blue. This is readily noted in plants and in low and high forms of animal life. In human beings red tends to raise blood pressure, pulse rate, respiration, and skin response (perspiration) and to excite brain waves. There is noticeable muscular reaction (tension) and greater frequency of eye blinks. Blue tends to have reverse effects, to lower blood pressure and pulse rate. Skin response is less, and brain waves tend to decline. The green region of the spectrum is more or less neutral. Reactions to orange and yellow are akin to reactions to red but less pronounced. Reaction to purple and violet is similar to reaction to blue. Psychological and psychic reactions to color are discussed in Chapters IV and VI.

To this writer the psychological aspects of color are more fascinating than the physiological. Proper colors for man-made environments are assuming vital importance. Many diseases of the body are being relieved and cured through modern medical practice, surgery, chemicals, and antibiotics, but "diseases" of the mind are very difficult to treat, and they are becoming more widespread in life today. As Carl Jung sagely observed in *The Integration of the Personality*, "The gigantic catastrophes that threaten us are not elemental happenings of a physical or biological kind, but are psychic events. . . . Instead of being exposed to wild beasts, tumbling rocks, and inundating waters, man is exposed today to the elementary forces of his own psyche."

As to the future, the vital importance of light—and color—to human survival is obvious enough. People in generations to come will no doubt travel into space and spend time there. They will live under the sea and within domed cities. Life will be very complicated—and artificial. Man's environment will be removed from nature, and he must master it or perish. Even now people young and old are spending increased amounts of time in schools, offices, hospitals, and institutions, with exposure to natural daylight ever less frequent.

Man is polluting and despoiling his natural environment. With his chemicals he is upsetting many of nature's balances. Mountains of waste are piling up everywhere and are being dumped into the sea and buried in caves. Man has even begun to fill the heavens with spent satellites, turning space beyond the clouds into the semblance of a used-car lot. He won't have to destroy himself in an instant with a hydrogen bomb: he will slowly choke himself to death.

Yet the age-old dream of harmony between nature and man forever ends in a collision between the two. Man must do penance for his sins against nature, but for his own survival he must be independent of the natural world. A scientist proclaims that, if man continues to denude the land of verdure, he will deprive the atmosphere of oxygen and all humanity will suffocate. Man, however, can make his own oxygen. For that matter, he can make his own food under artifical light and with fertilizers of his own concoction.

Nearly all human effort seems to be leading toward the controlled environment. It is inconceivable that this trend can be reversed or stopped. Nature is being left out in the country where man has more or less decided that she belongs. The mountains and seashore are becoming no longer the habitat of man but simply places for him to visit on weekends and holidays. Man thinks that he is too busy to be discommoded by nature. He has things to do in a hurry and cannot submit to anything capricious, natural or otherwise. It is wholly possible that within not too many decades man will venture from his contrived abodes into the vast stretches of nature, point through the clear plastic shell of his conveyance, and say to his children, "This may be hard to believe, but your ancestors used to live out there!"

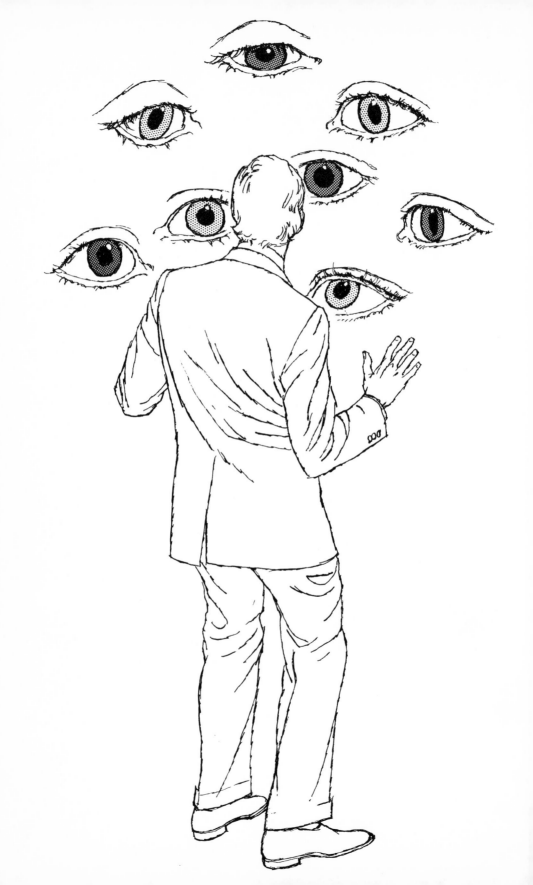

III. Visual Response

There is a great amount of mysticism and symbolism related to the human eye. The sun, for example, was the eye of god. The ancient Egyptian god Ra, driven from the earth by evil men, took refuge as the sun and thereafter peered down upon mankind's habits and peccadillos. The famous eye of Horus, who was son of Osiris and Isis, was symbolized in an amulet that is still worn as a bit of precious jewelry. Eyes have been painted on the prows of ships and airplanes. The curse of the evil eye has been countered with precious stones and red spots painted on foreheads.

Physiologically rather than mystically considered, the eye as a sense organ has had an engaging history. Early Greek Pythagorean theory (sixth century B.C.) held that visual rays were emitted by the eye, struck an object, and were reflected back. It was assumed that "fire" was within the eye. This could be observed if pressure was applied to the eye, as it caused the fire to flash. Such fire, like that of a torch, beacon, or lantern, was the active force of vision. This theory did not overlook the fact that sunlight illuminated the earth during the day, while night covered it in darkness. The fire of the eye simply supplemented natural light and cast special rays wherever vision was concentrated.

Plato wasn't too sure of this and spoke of a two-way phenomenon. "Let us carry out the principle . . . that nothing is self-existent, and that we shall see that every color, white, black, and every other color, arises out of the eye meeting the appropriate motion, and that what we term the substance of each color is neither the active nor passive element, but something which passes between them, as is peculiar to each percipient."

Aristotle denied that the eye contained fire. His successor, Theophrastus (fourth century B.C.), however, seemed to refer back to the ideas of Plato and Pythagoras but with qualifications. There probably were emissions from the eye. In talking of dizziness Theophrastus noted that a person might tremble and quiver while looking down from great heights. What happened here was that vision was set into distressing motion, which in turn upset the inner organs of the body. Yet upon looking into the sky no such strain occurred because empty distance simply absorbed the rays that came from the eye. "A stronger light extinguishes a weaker."

It was not until centuries later (sixteenth century A.D.) that the truer physiology of vision was revealed and the science of ophthalmology founded as it is known today. Precisely how color vision operates is still a mystery, and a fully acceptable theory or explanation has yet to be submitted by science.

EYELESS SIGHT

Before delving into the more reasonable aspects of vision and color vision and discussing modern viewpoints, let me tell of a few strange if not mystical curiosities.

In 1924 the French author Jules Romains published a book with the subtitle *Eyeless Sight*. While he never did enlist the support of the French Academy of Sciences, the success of his experiments was affirmed by many famous technical experts and scholars, among them Anatole France, who stoutly defended the theories of Romains. According to the Frenchman, the skin of man was sensitive to light (a fact that is certainly true of virtually all forms of life, man included). This he called paroptic perception. Using specially designed screens so that light would reach various parts of the body—but not the eyes—he stimulated paroptic perception to action. I quote from Romains' book: "For example, if the hands are bare, the sleeves lifted to the elbows, the forehead clear, the chest uncovered, the subject reads easily at a normal speed, a page of a novel or an article in a newspaper, printed in ordinary print."

Romains declared the hands to be most sensitive, then the neck and throat, cheeks, forehead, chest, back of neck, arms, and thighs. Elemental images formed in the tactile nerves "saw" color as well as form. He explains, "Our experiments place beyond doubt the existence in man of a *paroptic function*, that is, a function of visual perception of exterior objects (color and form), without the intervention of the ordinary mechanism of vision through the eyes." He contended that any intelligent person might be able to read the titles of a newspaper while blindfolded. "Under normal illumination the qualitative perception of colors is perfect." One might even "smell" colors through one's nose. "Perception of colors by the nasal mucosa is not of an olfactory order; that is, it does not consist in a recognition of *odors* belonging to the coloring substances. It is a perception specifically optical."

Not much progress was made for some time after Romains, for the world in which he lived was an incredulous one that demanded facts more substantial than the ones presented. About 40 years later a fabulous lady (then others) was found who could read and distinguish colors with the tips of her fingers. This revived fascination with the phenomenon, and it gained international publicity.

An excellent account of modern eyeless sight is given in the Sheila Ostrander and Lynn Schroeder book *Psychic Discoveries Behind the Iron Curtain.* A Russian girl, Rosa Kuleshova, could see with her fingers! Doubting doctors witnessed her ability to read type and name colors "as if she's grown a second set of eyes in her fingertips." Rosa was taken to Moscow, where she continued to perform wonders under close scrutiny. She still could "see" red, green, blue when the colored sheets were covered with tracing paper, cellophane, or glass. The great Russian Biophysics Institute of the Academy of Sciences was bewildered but had to admit Rosa's "dermo-optics." *Life* magazine at the time sent a reporter to Moscow and later ran an illustrated feature story.

Others appeared who had the same mystical ability, including a woman from Flint, Michigan, Mrs. Patricia Stanley. It seemed that some colors were sticky, some smooth, some rough. As she noted in *Life* magazine (June 12, 1964): "Light blue is smoothest. You feel yellow as very slippery, but not quite as smooth. Red, green, and dark blue are sticky. You feel green as stickier than red, but not as coarse. Navy blue comes over as the stickiest, and causes a braking feeling. Violet gives a greater braking effect that seems to slow the hand and feels even rougher."

There is a relationship here to eidetic imagery (discussed below): eyeless sight seems to be a natural endowment, for it is most noticeable in children from the ages of seven to twelve years. Could the blind be trained to see and distinguish colors with fingers, elbow, tongue, nose? Since Rosa Kuleshova the Russians have further investigated skin sight in the hopes that the blind could be given at least some "visual" perception, even if weak. A few have been so trained. Perhaps as long as the true organ of perception is in the brain, not in the eye, clues from the body, the skin can be used by the blind to "see" the world and its spectral hues. As Ostrander and Schroeder note, "If certain critical objects like doorknobs, faucets, telephones, handles on pots, dishes, particularly movable objects were colored, say, yellow in a room brilliantly lit with yellow bulbs, the blind might actually be able to see with their skin almost as easily as we locate a coffeepot with our eyes."

ABOUT "THOUGHTOGRAPHY"

Edward W. Russell in his *Design for Destiny* refers to a Professor T. Fukurai of Kohyassan University who "found that certain people can concentrate on design or picture and, by thought alone, transfer a clear reproduction to a sealed photographic plate, without the aid of light or a lens." Impossible? There is a similar, well-documented case regarding a man from Chicago. Ted Serios was a poorly educated bellhop in Chicago in the early 40s. He was temperamental, perhaps a bit psychopathic, and he had a drinking problem.

Yet Ted Serios could stare into a Polaroid camera and out would come (at times) vague photographs, less of people than places and structures such as the Eiffel Tower, Taj Mahal, White House. Dr. Jule Eisenbud, a psychiatrist and fellow of the American Psychiatric Association, took Ted Serios under his wing, moved him to Denver, and for two years submitted the man to a series of experiments that were in time witnessed by dozens of friends, scientists, photographers, and magicians. The result was an illustrated book of 368 pages by Jule Eisenbud (see the bibliography). A skeptical person might bring his own Polaroid camera, his own film, hold the device himself, and even trip the shutter, and out would come (not always, unfortunately) phantom prints of windmills, ships, automobiles, the Hilton Hotel in Denver, the tower of Westminster Abbey or a double-deck English bus.

Ted Serios could not explain his talent, nor did he have any interest in attempting to do so. He said that the gift would pass, and in time it did. In his fascinating book Jule Eisenbud comments, "Dr. Hans Berger, the discoverer of brain waves, granted the possible reality of telepathic communication but did not believe that whatever type of brain wave 'radiation' was measured by the EEG could account for them."

EIDETIC IMAGERY

To continue with the more mysterious aspects of vision, I shall now discuss the phenomenon of eidetic imagery. In recent years the study of vision and mental imagery has led to the discovery of numerous and astonishing phenomena. Among them is the magic of color that usually accompanies LSD. But first let us consider the better-known evidence of eidetic imagery in certain gifted individuals.

According to E. R. Jaensch in his book *Eidetic Imagery*, the images experienced by humans fall into three types—memory images, afterimages, and eidetic images. The first of these is the product of mind and imagination and has the quality of an idea or thought. The afterimage is more literal. It is actually seen and may have shape, design, dimension, and precise hue. Its size will vary as the eye gazes at near or far surfaces. It is generally a complementary image: white is seen in an area that was originally black, red is replaced by green, and so on. The third type, the eidetic image, is the most remarkable. Jaensch writes: "Eidetic images are phenomena that take up an intermediate position between sensations and images. Like ordinary physiological afterimages, they are always *seen* in the literal sense. They have this property of necessity under all conditions and share it with sensations."

Eidetic imagery is the gift of childhood, youth, the insane, the mystically inspired. While it is seemingly akin to the supernatural, it is nonetheless a sensory reality. The child playing with his toys may be able to project living pictures of them in his mind. These may not be mere products of the imagination. They may be far more tangible, with dimension, color, movement in their makeup. They are "lantern-slides" of the eye and brain, projected into definite, localized space. They are images as real as projected lantern-slides, and eye movements will follow their details. People in a hysterical state due to drugs or mental aberrations may find themselves attacked by ghoulish adversaries. Some have been known to run for their lives and even leap from windows. To some in the grip of delirium tremens rats have crept out of walls, and wires have projected from fingertips.

For the most part the phenomenon was given little attention until recent years. Because it vanishes with age and is likely to disappear at puberty, the adult mind, although capable of dealing with it, relegates it to the fervid period of childhood. Nevertheless images are seen. Pictures stand before the eyes, and details are distinguished in them that may be counted and identified in hue.

According to Jaensch, eidetic images are subject to the same laws as other sensations and perceptions. They are "in truth, merely the most obvious sign of the structure of personality normal to youth." Through them science might find plausible explanations for the reports of saints that walk out of pictures, of weird creatures, ghouls, and demons seen by human eyes. Because eidetic images are real sensations, ghouls and demons may also be real, and, instead of singing incantations and prescribing mental tests, the confessed observer might be treated as a sane human with a visual acuteness beyond the common stamp. Ghosts may live in heads rather than in old houses or castles.

For most persons there is an admitted gap between sensation and imagery, but as Jaensch claims, "Some people have peculiar 'intermediate experiences' between sensations and images." They are true eidetics whose responses are quite frank and spontaneous. To them sensation and imagination may go hand in hand and be closely united in some literal and graphic visual experience.

The phenomenon of eidetic imagery has much novelty and charm. In a more practical light, however, it may serve useful ends. Jaensch writes, "The eidetic investigators have already shown that the closest resemblance to the mind of the child is not the mental structure of the logician, but that of the artist." In education the forcing of an adult viewpoint, mind, and manner upon a child may suppress the eidetic personality and consequently may stand in the way of creative and natural expression. "For example, an eidetic child may, without special effort, reproduce symbols taken from the Phoenician alphabet, Hebrew words, etc. Or a person with a strong eidetic imagery may look at a number of printed words for a while and then go to the dark room and revive the text eidetically. It is possible to photograph the eye-movements occurring during the reading of the eidetic text."

HALLUCINOGENIC DRUGS

In the 60s a widespread drug cult was based on the simple foundation of a drop of lysergic acid diethylamide (LSD) on a lump of sugar. Across the nation countless persons, mostly young, suddenly swallowed the lump of sugar and took celestial trips, one of the most notable features of which was an explosion of brilliant, flowing, and flashing color the likes of which had never been witnessed on earth. In effect, the amazing discovery was made that a fantastic world of color existed within the human psyche. It lay buried as if in a golden cask, and a drop of LSD opened it up and let its magic burst forth. The process of vision was reversed—it came from inside out, not from the outside in.

How was science to explain this? While youths by the thousand lay on bare or carpeted floors and took acid trips—bum ones or grand ones— the medical profession diligently sought applications of the wonder drug. It had possibilities in some mental cases. It could be used to create states of euphoria in terminal cases. It could wipe out fear of death. It was, in effect, mind-expanding. It was inexpensive and amazingly potent: an eyedropper full of LSD was enough for 5,000 trips.

Hallucinogenic drugs had been known for centuries to exist in hashish, opium, peyote, mescal. Derived from cactus, the American Indian took peyote as part of religious ritual. The LSD cult in America during the 60s also frequently used it for religious purposes—to achieve harmony with all that was infinite. How to describe the effects of LSD? Aldous Huxley wrote, "Mescaline raises all colors to a higher power and makes the percipient aware of innumerable fine shades of difference, to which, at ordinary times, he is completely blind," Heinrich Kluver declared, "It is impossible to find words to describe mescal colors." Visions often have an oriental quality, like oriental rugs come to life but with colors of fabulous intensity.

One outstanding authority on LSD is Stanislav Grof. He has been chief of psychiatric research at the Maryland Psychiatric Research Center in Baltimore and assistant professor of psychiatry at Johns Hopkins University. Dr. Grof has done experimental work with LSD for over 15 years and has conducted over 2,000 psychedelic sessions. In *Psychiatry and Mysticism* (edited by Stanley R. Dean) he devotes a remarkable chapter to many of his observations. LSD trips can be down as well as up. There can on the one hand be feelings of cosmic unity, holiness, peace, bliss, and on the other hand extreme terror.

Grof offers many fascinating references to the experiences of different individuals. There can be cosmic engulfment, feelings of evil, persecution, with visions of dragons, pythons, octupuses: "A cosmic maelstrom sucking the subject and his world relentlessly to the center." There can be concepts of hell, unbearable suffering, war, epidemic, catastrophe. There can be death and rebirth, the release of great energy, with visions of explosions, volcanoes, atom bombs. There can be total annihilation, ego death. There can also be an overwhelming feeling of love. "The universe is perceived as indescribably beautiful." There can be "Visions of radiant sources of light experienced as divine, of a heavenly blue color, of a rainbow spectrum, of peacock feathers."

To bear out Jung's theory of the collective unconscious, some takers of LSD may witness their own birth and delivery from their mother's womb. There can be echoes of Greek mythology, biblical stories, pagan ceremonies. There can be ancestral throwbacks in which a person relives the experiences of his progenitors. There can be face-to-face meetings with the deities of old—Isis, Mazda, Apollo, Jehovah, Christ. Writes Grof, "The encounter with these deities is usually accompanied by very powerful emotions, ranging from metaphysical horror to ecstatic rapture."

Grof's interest lies in using LSD to treat various emotional disorders, schizophrenia, sexual deviation, alcoholism, drug addiction. His sessions, however, have also included scientists, philosophers, artists, educators. The taking of LSD has led to new art forms. In addition to brilliant colors, visions often reveal wavy lines, mosaics, flowers, animals, geometric patterns, jewels, gratings, lattices, honeycombs, fretwork, all of which tend to be animate. Artists have attempted to put these visions on canvas.

Out of the LSD cult came the discothèque of the late 60s and early 70s. Reversing the procedure of psychochemical ingestion, psychedelic discotheques using flashing lights, flowing colors, fluid designs and patterns, and roaring sounds attempted with fair success to blank out the real world for one of psychic and nightmarish fancy—without taking drugs. Flashing lights have been found to induce seizures of epilepsy, while pulsating, stroboscopic flashes may be hypnotic and produce headaches, nausea, and minor forms of a nervous breakdown.

AND NOW—BACK DOWN TO EARTH!

I will not attempt to describe the human eye or the process of vision but will concentrate on the subject of this chapter—visual response. James P. C. Southall has written: "Good and reliable eyesight is a faculty that is acquired only by a long process of training, practice and experience. Adult vision is the result of an accumulation of observations and associations of ideas of all sorts and is therefore quite different from the untutored vision of an infant who has not yet learned to focus and adjust his eyes and to interpret correctly what he sees. Much of our young lives is unconsciously spent in obtaining and coordinating a vast amount of data about our environment, and each of us has to learn to use his eyes to see just as he has to learn to use his legs to walk and his tongue to talk."

In Chapter II on biological response references are made to the role of light—and vision—in assuring the proper welfare and functioning of living things, man included. Light, of course, is essential to seeing, but its importance extends beyond this. For years the lighting industry was concerned chiefly with vision. Which lighting sources were most economical? Which gave the most light? In man's development since the beginning of time his light sources were the sun and sky, then firelight, the oil lamp, tallow candle, kerosene lamp, the carbon-filament lamp of Thomas Edison, mercury, sodium vapor, fluorescence, and others. The literature of the profession was dominated by references to recommended footcandles of light energy—*any light energy*—to enable men to see clearly at given tasks. As a consequence efficient light sources involving sodium or mercury vapor, fluorescent and other materials were developed and widely applied as if the only function of illumination was to enable man to see. This is no criticism. As long as man could walk into the open, play softball, swim, sit on the beach half-naked, all was well, for he could absorb the healthful rays of sunlight and keep in fair shape. But if man is to be confined for long hours, kept out of nature and away from the sun, he will need balanced light that emits a full or fairly full spectrum, including some ultraviolet. There is plenty of evidence that prolonged exposure to sodium or mercury vapor or to conventional fluorescent light will throw his system out of kilter.

In a specious way it could be argued that, given adequate diet and exercise, man could *survive* in total darkness. The blind man's world is dark only visually, for his body still absorbs radiant energy. If man does not live by bread alone, however, neither does he live too well by bad light or no light. Prolonged exposure of animals such as mice to narrow bands of the spectrum has had inimical effects. Aside from the biological effects of light, however, man is a psychic creature as well as a physical one. Sensory deprivation, a topic to be discussed in Chapter VIII, can drive him mad or at least out of his better wits. Anyone suffering from lingering mental or emotional shock will eventully have physical ailments and a shortened life span.

RESPONSES TO COLORED LIGHT

Most artificial environments today expose people to unbalanced light sources. Incandescent light is almost completely lacking in ultraviolet wavelengths. The glass tubes of most fluorescent-lighting fixtures absorb and screen out ultraviolet. Some mercury sources, rich in ultraviolet, lack red and infrared frequencies. Clear mercury lighting is objectionable because of the distortion of colors in an environment and the ugly appearance of the human complexion.

Setting aside the biological aspects of light, how about human *visual* responses to colored light? Years ago M. Luckiesh pointed out that yellow is in the region of maximum selectivity, the brightest portion of the spectrum. It is without aberration (that is, the eye normally focuses it perfectly), and it is psychologically pleasing. By experiment Luckish also demonstrated that by filtering out blue and violet radiation in a mercury light (also in a tungsten lamp) visual acuity remained practically constant despite the reduced amount of light absorbed by the filter. This would mean that as far as visual acuity is concerned yellow has definite advantages. Sodium light, for example, is highly efficient, although its distortion of colors makes it impossible to use under many circumstances.

C. E. Ferree and Gertrude Rand placed yellow illumination at the top of the list, followed by orange-yellow, yellow-green, and green. Deep red, blue, and violet were least desirable. Blue, in fact, is very difficult for the eye to focus and will cause objects to appear blurred and surrounded by halos. Under extreme dark adaptation, however, the eye seems to have best acuity under red light. Red illumination has been widely used for instrument panels in airplanes, for control rooms on ships and submarines. It has little influence on the dark-adapted eye and is not in fact seen on the outer boundaries of the retina, where the cones are lacking. It is therefore suitable as a blackout illuminant and will fail to stimulate the eye except when its rays strike near the fovea.

LIGHTING FOR GOOD APPEARANCE

One naive assumption by many who are concerned with artificial-light sources is that they ought to be as close as possible to natural daylight. If the room or area demands accurate color discrimination, imitation natural daylight may be necessary. But let it be fully appreciated that such light sources are far from flattering to the human complexion, which will turn sallow and grayish under their influence. Indeed, the proverbial use of cosmetics (before the advent of green and blue eyeshadow and white lipstick) was to daub pink powder on the skin and to apply red rouge to the cheeks and lips—to accent what most women considered to be nature's intention. Researchers have also found that human memory of true complexion color is substantially on the pinkish side.

What is natural light, after all? Daylight varies from morning to noon to evening, from pink and orange to yellow, white, blue, and back again to the warm hues of sunset. All this is *natural* light. A. A. Kruithof of Holland some time ago noted the fact that at *low* levels of illumination the world looks "normal" if the tint of the light is warm. (Cool light at low levels makes things look eerie and unnatural.) As illumination increases in intensity, cooler light is needed to assure normal appearances.

For the sake of good appearance warm light should be used at low levels and cooler or whiter light at high levels. Some lamp manufacturers are aware of this. Incandescent bulbs and warm-white fluorescent tubes are noted as having "greater preference at lower levels," while cool

white, daylight, and color-corrected mercury lamps have "greater preference at higher levels." Candlelight, real or simulated, is notable for its
cozy, friendly, and intimate atmosphere. Cool daylight is recommended
at high levels for work tasks and for the sale of merchandise. A cocktail
lounge would suggest live ghouls and dead ghosts if it were illuminated
by dim blue or violet light, whereas a school classroom or office under
brilliant red or pink light would be visually and psychologically objectionable—just as there are objections to sodium-vapor light (yellowish)
or mercury (greenish) whenever and wherever human complexion and
appearance are judged.

ENVIRONMENTAL COLOR

Let us now shift from light and illumination to color and brightness as
applied to the areas and surfaces of man-made environments. M.
Luckiesh has written, "A visual task is inseparable from its environment. . . . High visibility, ease of seeing and good seeing conditions are
overwhelmingly the result of good brightness engineering." And by
brightness engineering is meant the control of color as it may be seen by
human eyes on walls, ceilings, floors, furnishings. Here human responses
are to be radically affected.

To go from mice to men, in a study performed for the U.S. Atomic
Energy Commission in 1968 J. F. Spalding and two other researchers
investigated the influence of visible colors on voluntary activity in albino
RF-strain mice. The rodents were placed in cubicles for periods of 18
hours, rested, and then placed for 18 hours in other cubicles until all
environments were tested. The measure of activity was determined by
the revolutions of activity wheels similar to those seen in squirrel cages.
Mice are nocturnal animals and hence are most active in darkness, as
results of the test showed. The next greatest activity was with red light.
The RF-strain mouse experiences red as darkness. "Activity in yellow
light was significantly greater than in daylight, green, blue and significantly less than in dark and red." Incidentally, blind mice showed little
difference in activity, regardless of color, bearing out the claim that
the effects discovered were "due to visual receptors."

Human responses to color in an environment will be further treated
in the next chapter on emotional response. It has often been assumed by
some technical minds in the field of vision that human beings see best and
are most comfortable in an environment in which all areas in the field of
view are of uniform brightness. Unfortunately, this not only is far from

the truth but is an inversion of fact. As is repeated elsewhere in this book, particularly in Chapter VIII, which deals with sensory deprivation, visual (and emotional) comfort demands constant change and variety. According to H. L. Logan, the human organism is in a constant state of flux. All its functions rise and ebb continually. Simple thoughts will affect respiration and pulse rate. So pronounced is this tendency for physiological and psychological experiences to fluctuate that they will take place even when the exterior world remains the same. Areas of steady brightness will appear to fade in and out. The pupil opening of the eye will actually close and dilate slightly. Steady sounds will not be heard consistently. Sensations of taste, heat, cold, and pressure will all vary and will be surprisingly independent of unvarying stimuli in the early stages of exposure. If the monotony is long continued, the ability to respond to the stimulus will deteriorate.

People require varying, cycling stimuli to remain sensitive and alert to their environments. Comfort and agreeableness are normally identified with moderate if not radical change, and this change concerns brightness as well as all other elements in the environment. If overstimulation may cause distress, so may severe monotony.

THE HAZARDS OF HIGH BRIGHTNESS

Glare is inimical not only to clear vision but to physical, mental, and emotional comfort. As a simple example, no doubt the reader has noted the distress that may accompany visual exposure to a snow-covered field *even on a cloudy day.* "Retinal injury has been known to occur in humans suffering from 'snowblindness,' the result of reflected sunlight," states T. R. C. Sisson.

White and off-white are popular finishes for walls in homes. I have no objection to this other than to say that white has little emotional appeal; it is neutral, sterile, and likely to be monotonous if not boring. Wide expanses of white aesthetically lend themselves to accent colors in furnishings, and this may be pleasing, but excessive use of white on walls (and also perhaps on ceilings, floors, and furnishings) in such places as offices, schools, and hospitals will lead to definite hazards *if this white environment also includes high levels of illumination.*

Classical work was done many years ago by C. E. Ferree and Gertrude Rand at the request of the American Medical Association. At the time they wrote: "The eye has grown up under daylight. Under this condition only three adjustments have developed, and indeed only three are needed: the reaction of the pupil to regulate the amount of light entering the eye and to aid the lens in focusing the light from objects at different distances, and accommodation and convergence to bring the object on the principal axis of the lens and the image on the fovea." These adjustments tended to be coordinated. When they were separated, trouble was encountered. High brightness in the field of view, if isolated from the task, might cause disruption. The eye would thereupon struggle to set things right. *"This striving to clear up its vision by ineffectual maladjustment is the cause of what is commonly called eyestrain."* As a further warning, Ferree and Rand concluded: "The presence of high brilliancies in the field of view produces a strong incentive for the eyes to fixate and accommodate for them, which incentive must be controlled by voluntary effort. The result of this opposition of voluntary control against strong reflex incentive is to tire the eye quickly and to make it lose the power to sustain the precision of adjustment needed for clear seeing of the work."

Ophthalmologists are in agreement here. White glare, as a form of artificial snow blindness, can cause congestions in the eye, inflammation, and scotoma. It can aggravate muscular imbalance, refractive difficulties, nearsightedness, and astigmatism—perhaps not in a day or week but over a prolonged period. Where difficult eye tasks are to be performed, high brightness in the general field of view puts seeing efficiency in reverse. That is, the eye is *quick* in adjusting to brightness and *slow* in adjusting to darkness. If the surround is bright and the task is dark, ability to work effectively will be seriously handicapped.

PRACTICAL APPLICATIONS

There are lessons to be learned from the above remarks. Many of the readers of this book may be architects, interior designers, decorators, and others concerned with the "functional" use of color in human habitats (homes excepted, where personal taste should probably dominate). On the matter of *brightness* behavior and attention may be easily directed through the principles described.

If attention is best directed *outward* toward an environment, perhaps in interiors where *muscular* work may be done and where hazards may exist, a bright environment (yellow, coral, orange) is recommended. Accompanied by plenty of light, the human eye will look at and adjust to its surroundings. Safety may be well served. If the interior is meant for more sedentary tasks, for severe use of the eye or mind, it will be best to reduce the brightness of the environment as a source of distraction. With walls, floors, equipment in medium tones (green, blue-green, beige, terracotta) and with extra light over tasks, if necessary, people will be better able to concentrate. It will be noted that in difficult mental tasks many will close their eyes to eliminate the environment completely. One advantage of these two principles is that they allow for a wide variety of color choices. Emphasis is on brightness, with the aesthetic factor of hue optional.

COLORED VISION

About eight percent of men have some color deficiency in vision, but less that one-half percent of women. The usual deficiency is to red or green or both. Brown and olive green, for example, may look the same.

There are instances where color blindness may be induced or where it may follow certain pathological conditions. Here are some examples. In jaundice the world may appear predominantly yellowish. Red vision may follow retinal hemorrhage or snow blindness. Yellow vision may follow digitalis or quinine poisoning. Green vision may be caused by wounds of the cornea. Blue vision has been reported in cases of alcoholism. In tobacco scotoma the vision may be reddish or greenish. In santonin poisoning the world may at first appear bluish. There may be a second stage of longer duration of yellow vision and a stage of violet sight before complete recovery. Following the extraction of a cataract the patient may experience red vision, sometimes followed by blue vision. Green and yellow are rare.

Vision and the organ of sight have been subjects of extensive medical research. In color therapy attempts have been made to relieve certain conditions of human distress by shining colors into the eye in an effort to stimulate or relax eye nerves and in turn to affect the body itself, possibly through a chain of interreactions. Blue and violet lights shining into the eye have been reported favorably in cases of headaches. Red light is said to increase blood pressure and cope with some types of dizziness. Yellow, green, or blue light is said to relieve digestive ills; yellow light, to be beneficial in certain cases of mental disorder.

These responses are elaborated upon in Chapter VII. If man is sensitive to color, so also does his body become a palette of hues. Arthur Abbott in his book *The Color of Life* gives an excellent description of the protean aspects assumed by the human body. "The redness of blood is influenced by oxygen and carbon dioxide. The rosy cheeks of youth indicate a healthy blood condition, together with a delicate and healthy skin. A white man can appear all colors under certain conditions, so he might more appropriately be called 'colored,' whereas the Negro, whom we speak of as 'colored,' is black, which denotes an absence of color. A white man can appear nearly white from fright, loss of blood, etc.; grayish from pain; red from exertion, anger, etc.; greenish from biliousness and introduced poisons; yellow from jaundice; blue from cold, poor circulation, and lack of oxygen; brown from sun tan; purple from strangulation; and black from decay."

VISION—NOT ALWAYS A BLESSING

I end this chapter on a dispiriting note. Poets have written on the blessings of sight. The Bible tells of vision restored to the blind. There have been many plots and plays in which a magnificent world of color has been revealed to the once sightless. Vision is surely one of life's greatest blessings. But the biblical parables, the dramatic legends and tales of restored sight do not invariably lead to boundless joy for those to whom vision has come again, miraculously or otherwise. R. L. Gregory writes in *Eye and Brain*, "Depression in people recovering sight after many years of blindness seems to be a common feature of the cases." He reports on one man of fifty-two who found difficulty in making an adjustment to sight after a successful corneal operation. What he had learned through the sense of touch apparently was contradicted when his vision was restored. "He found the world drab, and was upset by flaking paint and blemishes on things. He liked bright colors, but became depressed when the light faded. His depressions became marked and general. He gradually gave up active living, and three years later he died." Let me cheer my reader. There are happier responses to color to be described in the next chapter!

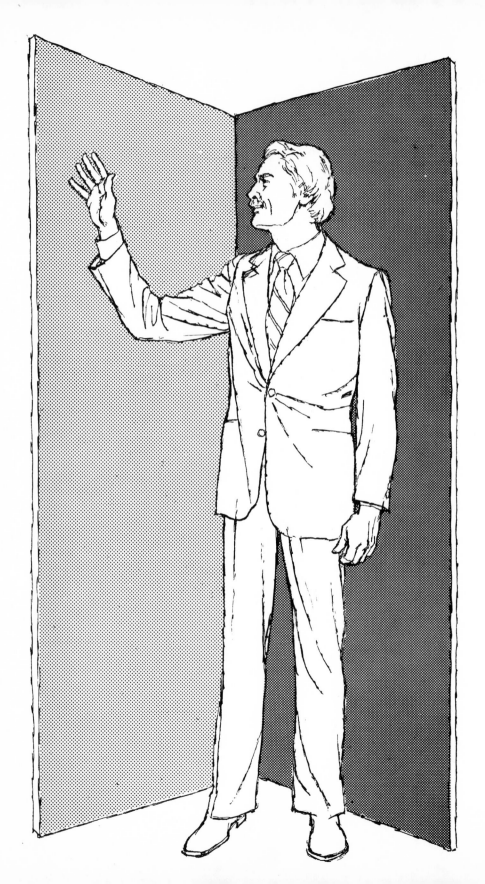

IV. Emotional Response

I have had considerable experience in the application of color to human environments but less in homes than in industries and institutions where work tasks are performed or where good visual, physical, and emotional wellbeing must be assured. While a number of clinical tests have been made, they have chiefly concerned eye fatigue and its effect on body and frame of mind. Ophthalmic instruments have been used to measure rate of eye blinks and retinal fatigue—with eye specialists called upon to check the need for medical treatment or corrective eyeglasses after specified periods of time.

Such testimony has been directly and simply acquired, for instruments can be used and factual data recorded. But in psychological realms the factual and "scientific" approach is not so easy. The bodies of people are very much the same, but their minds and spirits are radically different. Research in the field of psychology is always difficult. Conscious reactions to color or anything else are by no means necessarily the same as unconscious reactions, and the two may conflict. In art, for example, there are those who prefer realism and dislike the abstract and vice versa. Surely neither attitude is correct nor absolute as applied to *all* persons.

Are colors "warm" and "cool?" Some years ago a study was made in the lighting field with negative results, and the *Lighting Handbook* of the Illuminating Engineering Society declared, "This appears to have no foundation in fact." The word "fact" is forever a troublesome one in relation to anything emotional. The facts of hunger might be measured in terms of the flow of gastric juices in a person's stomach. But who would be *hungry* if some technician put a rubber tube into the stomach to extract the juices! The evidence of the senses must be accepted, facts or no facts. If red is a warm color to you and a cool one to me, such are facts but personal to each of us.

This chapter is concerned with emotional reactions to color. The studies presented and the results described are frankly subject to question and can be disputed. I present them anyhow, fully aware of the *fact* that if individual reactions differ, average reactions among groups of people can be justification enough to reach tolerable conclusions. All people do not have to accept red as a warm color, but if a majority of them do, this will suffice. Later chapters describe instruments (polygraph, EEG) used to record human responses to color. For the present let me describe experiments, old and new, relating to color and emotional response.

Emotional reactions to color may not be as vague and elusive as some have thought. They may have a physiological as well as a psychological basis. Kendric C. Smith, former president of the American Society for Photobiology, writes: "The psychological effects of light, particularly of colored light, are well known but not well understood. These effects may bear a causal relationship to purely biological processes in the brain induced by light, which in turn will affect psychic behavior. Light intensity as well as wavelength specificity may alter productivity and mood." John Ott further concurs, "Behind the psychological responses to color are more basis responses to specific wavelengths of radiant energy."

BACK INTO HISTORY

In 1875 a European doctor by the name of Ponza fitted several rooms with colored-glass windows, colored walls, and colored furnishings. Red and blue were the colors principally used. Regarding red ne wrote, "After passing three hours in a red room a man afflicted with taciturn delirium became gay and cheerful; on getting up the day after his entry into the room, another madman who had refused all food whatever asked for breakfast, and ate with surprising avidity." As to blue, "A violent case who had to be kept in a strait jacket was shut in the room with the blue window; less than an hour afterwards he had become calmer." Today, however, the red and blue rooms of the asylum are no more. The medical profession has applied new therapies, methods, equipment, drugs. The use of color, where specified for environments, has become quite sophisticated, as will be described in chapter VIII. Color, of course, is not a cure, but it serves a purpose in helping to inspire an agreeable mood in human beings—always essential to the best of medical care.

In 1910 Stein called attention to a general light tonus in the muscular reactions of the human body. The word "tonus" refers to the condition of steady activity maintained by the body. Conditions of muscular tension and muscular relaxation, for example, are tonus changes. They are to some extent noticeable and measurable and are a good clue to the action of color. Feré discovered that red increased muscular tension from a normal 23 units to 42. Orange increased the units to 35, yellow to 30, green to 28, and blue to 24—all above normal. In the main, however, the warm hues of the spectrum are stimulating, while the cool hues are relaxing.

Through optic excitation A. Metzger observed that, when light was thrown on one eye of many animals and humans, a tonus condition could be produced in the corresponding half of the body. Accompanying these tonus changes were changes in "the superficial and deep-seated sensation, both showing a regular dependence upon optical stimuli." He concluded that the influence of light acted not only on the muscles but was effective in producing changes throughout the entire organism.

As an experimental method Metzger had his subject stretch out his arms horizontally in front of his body. When light was thrown on one eye, there would be a tonus increase on the same side of the body. The arm on the side of the light would raise and deviate toward the side of the illuminated eye. When colors were employed, red light would cause the arms to spread away from each other. Green light would cause them to approach each other in a series of jerky motions. In cases of torticollis (twitching of the head) exposure to red light increased restlessness, while green light decreased it.

Equally interesting were the experiments of H. Ehrenwald. He demonstrated that, when the face and neck were illuminated from the side, the outstretched arms would deviate toward red light and away from blue. And this reaction took place independently of the sense of vision! It occurred when the eyes were sealed to light and had even been observed in blind individuals!

Tonus reflex seems to be in two directions, with yellow-green as the neutral point where no specific reaction takes place. Toward orange and red there is an attraction to stimulus. Toward green and blue there is a withdrawal from it. Even infrared and ultraviolet, both invisible, will cause reflex actions, lending further evidence to the fact that the body does react to color without even seeing it. While some later experimenters have found reason both to agree and disagree with Metzger and Ehrenwald, no one can doubt today that the human body responds to light and color and indeed that it also emits radiation on its own.

FELIX DEUTSCH

In 1937 Felix Deutsch, a physician, did commendable research on the emotional effects of color. His findings throw important light not only on medical practice with reference to color but on the whole psychology of color. Deutsch writes, "Every action of light has in its influence physical as well as psychic components." Simply stated, light energy affects the body directly and also through the eye and brain. He points out, for example, that in treatment of pulmonary diseases such as tuberculosis with light there is a true biological effect. Beyond this, however, the patient shows a cheerful response to the pleasing qualities of fresh air and sunshine. He experiences "sensations and psychic excitations, which, through the vegetative nervous system, boost all life functions: increase the appetite, stimulate circulation, etc., and through these manifestations the physical influence of light upon the disease process is in turn enhanced." Thus Deutsch speaks of a light influence and a light impression. The one is physical, the other emotional. Each is individually therapeutic, and both together comprise a highly efficacious "remedy" in a great many instances.

It is a matter of common observation that the moods of men are changed by environment, by ugliness and beauty, by sunny weather and rainy weather. Reactions to color are likewise depressing or inspiring. Placed in a bright, harmonious setting, most people will find their dispositions improved. And with a better spirit the vascular system, pulse, blood pressure, nervous and muscular tension may be favorably affected. These responses are subtle and do not follow any universal laws, according to Deutsch. "In estimating these reactions which one could also call emotional and which only secondarily show their manifestations organically, one has to rely almost exclusively upon the statements made by the individuals tested, statements whose validity is not always easy to determine."

This early work by Deutsch well anticipated similar confidence and optimism by other qualified and authoritative researchers who came after him. He wrote further: "The influence of mood, psychic disturbance, fear, happiness, sadness, and impressions from the outer world make themselves readily noticeable in both subjective and objective changes referable to the vascular system. Changes in pulse frequency and rhythm as well as fluctuations in blood pressure are objective expressions of the psychically influencing factors which have taken place." He treated patients whose conditions were of nervous origin or who had disturbances in heart rhythm. "During the period of investigation all other therapeutic measures which might have affected the vascular system were abandoned."

Deutsch's methods were far from superficial. A room was chosen overlooking a garden. The glass panes of the windows were arranged to accommodate different hues, and colored artificial light was employed in the interior. Two main colors were enlisted, a warm red and a cool green. The subject was asked to look quietly out the window. He was left alone for a quarter of or half an hour. After this he was questioned regarding his general feeling and about his impression of the illumination. Finally he was asked to build free associations and to recall anything that might have come to his mind.

Deutsch described a number of cases and the results that followed exposure to the colorful interiors. One patient troubled with anginal fear complained of shortness of breath, air hunger, and palpitation of the heart. She feared the return of a spasm that years ago had caused her to lose consciousness. In another case the patient complained of attacks of weakness, shortness of breath, and pressure sensations over the chest that led to fear of choking.

Deutsch studied and measured reductions in blood pressure and otherwise observed any changes or improvements in the physical health and mental wellbeing of his patients. He summarized his conclusions as follows. Color brings about a reflex action upon the vascular system, if only through the feelings and emotions. The effect achieved is not specific for any one or several hues. Warm colors may calm one person and excite another. Cool colors may likewise be stimulating to one person and passive to another. Irradiation with red or green light may produce an elevation of blood pressure and a quickening of pulse rate. Or the opposite may take place, depending on the particular psychic makeup of the individual.

What happens? According to Deutsch, "The emotional excitements which are recognized through changes in blood pressure, pulse-frequency and rhythm, are brought forth through association." Green may recall nature, mountains, lakes. Red may recall the sunset, the fireplace. "These superficial associations lead to deeper lying memories, which explain the affective emphasis of the attitudes toward the colors."

This summary is quite fair. It should be noted that Deutsch avoided making specific claims for specific colors—with which this author fully agrees. Color in itself, all colors, are psychologically therapeutic. "The psychic process which is brought into play here is easily stated: the colored light changes the environment. Through the changed appearance of the environment the individual is lifted out of reality." He is on the road to recovery, helped along by his own mental and emotional processes.

KURT GOLDSTEIN

Another stimulating writer and researcher has been Kurt Goldstein, who in his book *The Organism* and in many articles for the medical press has found therapeutic and psychotherapeutic values in color.

Goldstein writes, "It is probably not a false statement if we say that a *specific color stimulation is accompanied by a specific response pattern of the entire organism.*" Confirming the work of Metzger and Ehrenwald already mentioned, organic response may be noted when the stimulation of color is carefully introduced and its action observed. This would mean that response to color is deep-set, that it is entwined in the life process. "The influence of color is increased in neurotics and psychotics." Goldstein writes of a woman with a cerebellar disease who had a tendency to fall unexpectedly and to walk with an unsteady gait. When she wore a red dress, such symptoms were more pronounced. Green and blue clothing had an opposite effect and restored her equilibrium almost to normal.

Color may thus affect the ability of the body to maintain its position. As already stated, red light may cause the outstretched arms to spread away from each other; green light may cause them to move toward each other. In a patient with a left-sided lesion of the brain the arm on the affected side deviated far more than normal. "Because this deviation under certain conditions is definite in amount and is changed definitely by different color stimulations, this phenomenon can be used as an indicator in studying the influence of colors on performance."

The equilibrium of the human organism is disturbed far more by red than it is by green. Goldstein thus came to a conclusion that offers an important answer to those concerned with human response to color. He states: "The stronger deviation of the arms in red stimulation corresponds to the experience of being disrupted, thrown out, abnormally attracted to the outerworld. It is only another expression of the patient's feeling of obtrusion, aggression, excitation, by red. The diminution of the deviation [to green stimulation] corresponds to the withdrawal from the outerworld and retreat to his own quietness, his center. The inner experiences represent the psychological aspect of the reactions of the organism. We are faced in the observable phenomena with the physical aspect." Many persons suffering from tremors and twitching may find such disturbances relieved if green glasses are worn. They screen out red light rays and have a quieting effect.

As a generalization on the specification of color, perhaps for any facilities occupied by groups of persons at work or under medical or psychological treatment, Goldstein offers this intriguing prescription: "One could say *red is inciting to activity and favorable for emotionally-determined actions; green creates the condition of meditation and exact fulfillment of the task. Red may be suited to produce the emotional background out of which ideas and action will emerge; in green these ideas will be developed and the actions executed*" [Goldstein's emphasis].

CECIL STOKES—COLOR AND MUSIC

There are strong emotional relationships between color and music, and many have written about it. While any *physical* relationship (frequency of vibrations) can be doubted, a feeling of harmony between music and color is quite universal. Wagner wrote about it as a composer, and Kandinsky wrote about it as an artist—among many other artists and observers.

Around 1921 Thomas Wilfred developed an art of mobile color which he called lumia. Wilfred, however, had little interest in anything therapeutic. Later in the 40s Cecil Stokes of California was able to apply abstract color-and-sound motion-picture films to the treatment of psychotic patients. Cecil Stokes was born in England on April 6, 1910 and died at the age of 46 in Los Angeles on December 14, 1956. During his life he directed the Auroratone Foundation of America in Hollywood and was able to establish a number of sanctuaries of music and color in government hospitals throughout America. Stokes was one of the forerunners of later light festivals, electric circuses, and discothèques in which dynamic light patterns, sound-induced colors, electronic gadgets, and bizarre films and projections assault the senses to ends that he himself understood all too well over three decades ago.

Cecil Stokes created and engineered what became known as Auroratone films. Abstract mobile patterns *in full color* covered a broad screen to the accompaniment of music—André Kostalanetz and his orchestra playing *Clair de Lune*, Bing Crosby singing *Home on the Range, Going My Way, Ave Maria*. The color effects were derived from growing and expanding crystal formations photographed in Technicolor with polarized light (a technique that is well known today). In any event the colors flowed gracefully and majestically before the eyes in delightful and totally natural patterns. Through some skill known only to Stokes the tempo of pattern change and the crescendo and diminuendo of color intensity were remarkably harmonized with the visual and emotional qualities of the music.

The work of Stokes was nicely documented in an article by Herbert E. Rubin and Elias Katz that includes two full-page, full-color frames from one of the films. Rubin and Katz set about to "observe the effects of Auroratone films on psychotic depressions . . . to explore the psychodynamics underlaying the reactions of psychotic depressed patients when exposed to these films, and to use these films as a psychotherapeutic agent." The article presented in detail the results of the study and quoted from six case reports. "It was noted that manic-depressives in the depressed state had catharsis experiences and appeared to benefit from exposure to the films."

As explained by Rubin and Katz, a badly injured or crippled patient may become seriously depressed. He may stubbornly resist medical aid and strive to commit suicide. As the depression grows worse, he may become tragically ill. With the prescription of music and color as in the Auroratone films, however, "Most patients become more accessible. . . . Those whose speech was previously blocked or retarded, spoke more freely. . . . In this state of accessibility it was possible for the psychiatrist to establish rapport."

If the discothèques and rock-and-roll bands, with their strobe lights, flashing colors, and screeching sounds, put nerves on edge, break through human timidity and inhibitions, stimulate effects similar to those that follow the taking of LSD, if they cause minor forms of a nervous breakdown, Cecil Stokes had precisely opposite hopes for his sound-color medium. With "slow, sedative and mildly sad music," he was sure that mentally ill souls "could ventilate their pent-up tensions resulting from conflicts and frustrations." He was concerned as a pioneer with psychic and psychological values in color and sound, with environmental influences and controls that will undoubtedly be further developed and more widely applied as time goes on.

Here is an abstract of one case from the Rubin and Katz article: "Patient E. This 26-year-old patient was admitted . . . on 5 June 1945 for further treatment of multiple second and third degree burns of the body. . . . He did not show any mental symptoms until 16 August 1945 when he wrote on American Red Cross stationery, 'Please get some poison to kill me.' The patient is disfigured as a result of severe burns of the face involving the ears as well as both hands. He is restless, agitated, depressed, retarded and self-absorbed. He ruminates a great deal about having lost his grip on life. . . . He frequently expresses a desire to die as a means of solving his emotional problem. . . . 21 September 1945. Prior to the showing the patient appeared somewhat depressed. He sat with his head down and fumbled with his shoes. Throughout the showing, he seemed completely absorbed with the music and the color. . . . At the close of the showing, he sat up and looked about the room. His countenance was no longer despondent. During the group discussion afterward, he cooperated with the psychiatrist, answering questions freely. As he left the room he did not drag his feet."

BLUE IS BEAUTIFUL

This is the title of a short article that appeared in the September 17, 1973 issue of *Time* magazine. Reference was made to the work of Henner Ertel, director of an institute for rational psychology at Munich. A three-year study was conducted among children to judge, if not measure, the impact of environmental color on learning capacity. Rooms with low ceilings were painted in different colors. The better and more popular colors were light blue, yellow, yellow-green, and orange. In these environments IQ could be raised as much as 12 points. So-called ugly colors—white, black, brown—caused a drop in IQ. "Researchers found that the popular colors also stimulated alertness and creativity; white, black and brown playrooms made children duller." These findings by Ertel confirm this writer's objection to white, gray, or colorless walls in any interiors where groups of persons are assembled and where physical comfort, visual efficiency, manual skill, and emotional poise are to be promoted. Ertel found the color orange to improve social behavior, to cheer the spirit, and lessen traits of hostility and irritability, a finding that this writer has confirmed.

Adjustment to environment is no doubt the beginning of awareness and understanding for all animals, man included. Most people have witnessed or seen in motion pictures the birth of chickens, calves, colts. First there is curiosity about the world about them, followed by a close attachment to the protection of the mother. Henner Ertel and his associates, with this observation in mind, designed a plexiglass crib to enable the newborn to see what was going on around them. For a number of infants so reared mental development was aided. "At 18 months, children in the experimental group were measurably more intelligent than two-year-olds who have been confined to traditional cribs." Environmental color recommendations drawn from my experience are presented in Chapter VIII.

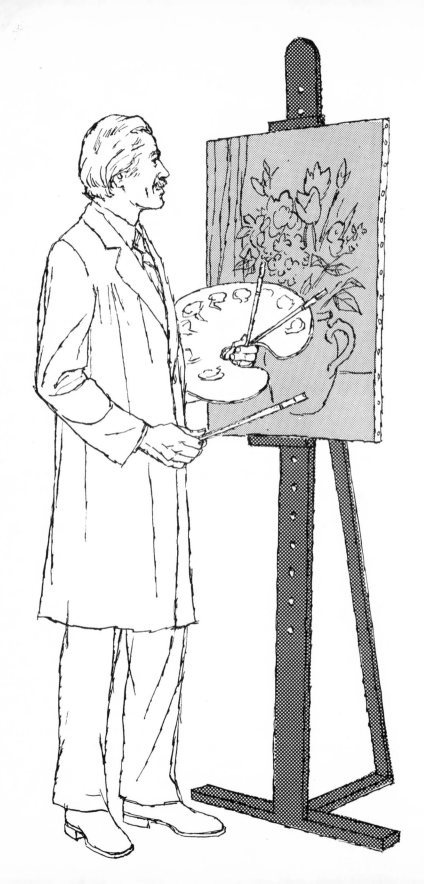

V. Aesthetic Response

Many books have been written on the subject of this chapter. Principles of color harmony have been of interest not only to artists but to architects, designers, workers in textiles, ceramics, glass, mosaics—and gardeners and flower arrangers. There is much repetition on the theme of concordant color combination. There are color circles, color scales, gadgets with masks and dials. And there are innumerable references to the individual feelings and theories of individual artists.

SYMBOLISM VS PERSONAL EXPRESSION

It is well to make clear that early man's use of color was not essentially concerned with aesthetics. Today's attitude toward color as a thing of beauty dates more or less from the Renaissance, not before. To early man there were beauty and glory in color and design. But his expression in art was not prompted by an aesthetic or emotional urge so much as by a consuming desire to symbolize the mysteries of the universe and the powers of the supernatural. Egyptian hieroglyphics and tomb and coffin decorations were not precious ornaments for delicate tastes. Speaking of the Egyptian vignettes found in the *Book of the Dead* E. A. Wallis Budge says: "It is possible that they may have been added merely as illustrations of the various texts of that work, but I believe that, like the drawings of the Bushmen which are found in caves in South Africa, they were drawn and painted with an object that had nothing to do with artistic ideas or development. That object was to benefit the dead by magical means." And the same was true in the embellishment of interiors, in sculpture, painting, design—not only in the valley of the Nile but in Chaldee, in India, China, Greece, and Rome! With his wall decorations, statues, vignettes man charmed his existence, worshipped his gods, portrayed his philosophy and science, identified every quarter of the earth and the heavens, recorded his history, protected his life, and assured his salvation.

During some 4,000 years up to the time of the Renaissance the palette of color was as simple as described in Chapter I—red, gold, yellow, green, blue, purple, black, white. No doubt such colors were simple because they were tokens of man's knowledge and philosophy. They spoke of the mysteries, of gods, devils, immortality. In consequence they were vigorous and brilliant. Only red—not pink or old rose or maroon—could stand for mankind, the element fire, the hue of day. Only blue—neither tinted nor shaded—could represent the element air, the hue of God the Father. The colors had to be direct because they gave direct and vivid interpretations of life on earth and in the hereafter.

Much of this ancient symbolism is given in Chapter I of this book. What is quite remarkable is that virtually the same palette of colors is found in all old civilizations from Africa to Asia Minor, Asia, Europe, and the Mayans and Incas of North and South America. As to Greek architecture and sculpture (most of which was colored, by the way), the same few colors were used over and over and again and again for centuries. While some fairly realistic portraits have been found, none of the ancient artists (mostly anonymous) ever indulged in abstract or purely romantic expression—i.e., the "spirit" of anything such as freedom, hope, charity, inspiration—which has delighted so many artists of modern times. Indeed, these early decorators were concerned with practical matters such as harmony with nature and the gods, pleas for rain, good harvests, relief from plague and disease, life after death.

DA VINCI AND THE RENAISSANCE

Let me begin my story of modern concepts of color harmony with Leonardo da Vinci, who wrote eloquently and with great insight in his *A Treatise on Painting*. Long before the days of photography he declared: "The first aim of the painter is to make it appear that a round body in relief is presented upon the flat surface of his picture; and he who surpasses others in this respect, deserves to be esteemed more skillful than they in his calling. Now this perfection of art comes from the true and natural arrangement of light and shade, or what is called chiaroscuro; thus if a painter dispenses with shadows when they are necessary, he wrongs himself and renders his work despicable to connoisseurs, to win the worthless applause of the vulgar and ignorant, who look only at the brilliance and gaiety of the color in a picture, and care nothing for the relief."

Da Vinci had definite ideas about color, beauty, and harmony. Rather than interpret his views, I shall let him speak for himself. "Of different bodies equal in whiteness, and in distance from the eye, that which is surrounded by the greatest darkness will appear the whitest; and on the contrary, that shadow will appear the darkest which has the brightest white round it.

"Of different colors equally perfect, that will appear most excellent which is seen near its direct contrary: a pale color against red; a black upon white . . . blue near yellow; green near red: because each color is more distinctly seen, when opposed to its contrary, than to any other similar to it."

"If you mean to represent great darkness, it must be done by contrasting it with great light; on the contrary, if you want to produce great brightness, you must oppose to it a very dark shade: so a pale yellow will cause red to appear more beautiful than if opposed to a purple color.

"There is another rule, by observing which, though you do not increase the natural beauty of the colors, yet by bringing them together they may give additional grace to each other, as green placed near red, while the effect would be quite the reverse, if placed near blue.

"Harmony and grace are also produced by a judicious arrangement of colors, such as blue with pale yellow or white, and the like."

As to his painting methods: "After black and white comes blue and yellow, then green and tawny or umber, and then purple and red. These eight colors are all that nature produces. With these I begin my mixtures, first black and white, black and yellow, black and red; then yellow and red." To this he adds, "Black is more beautiful in the shades; white in the strongest light; blue and green in the half tint; yellow and red in the principal light; gold in the reflexes; and lake in the half-tint."

Da Vinci's style of painting (chiaroscuro) dominated the Renaissance and following generations. He understood colored shadows, conjoined shadows, cast shadows. Perhaps he anticipated abstract art when he wrote: "By throwing a sponge impregnated with various colors against a wall, it leaves some spots upon it, which may appear like a landscape. It is true also, that a variety of compositions may be seen in such spots, according to the disposition of mind with which they are considered; such as heads of men, various animals, battles, rocky scenes, seas, clouds, woods, and the like." Da Vinci favored knowledge and understanding against mere feeling. "Whoever flatters himself that he can retain in his memory all the effects of nature, is deceived, for our memory is not so capricious: therefore consult nature for everything."

SIR JOSHUA REYNOLDS

All artists of modern times have had strong feelings about color, and all have prided themselves on unusual talent in their color expression. I prefer to devote the rest of this chapter to fairly knowledgeable and original theories of color harmony, with a brief interlude for Sir Joshua Reynolds. He wrote: "It ought, in my opinion, to be indispensably observed that the masses of light in a picture be always of a warm mellow color, yellow, red, or a yellowish-white; and that the blue, the gray, or the green colors be kept almost entirely out of these masses, and be used only to support and set off these warm colors; and for this purpose a small portion of cool colors will be sufficient. Let this conduct be reversed; let the light be cold and the surrounding colors warm, as we often see in the works of the Roman and Florentine painters, and it will be out of the power of art, even in the hands of Rubens or Titian, to make a picture splendid and harmonious." Reynolds apparently felt very sure of his generalization. It is said that Gainsborough deliberately refuted and reversed the principle and in so doing painted his well-known masterpiece, *The Blue Boy*.

JOHANN WOLFGANG VON GOETHE

The great German poet Goethe devoted many years to the study of color and took bitter exception to the scientific theories of Newton. Here, however, Goethe was in error. What he contributed to the art of color was the enthusiasm, spirit, and remarkable insight of a genius. He devised color circles and triangles.

Goethe had strong opinions about aesthetic and emotional factors in color. He believed that all colors derived from lightness and darkness and that the two basic primaries were yellow and blue. Some colors were "plus"—yellow, red-yellow (orange), yellow-red (cinnabar). As to yellow: "In its highest purity it always carries with it the nature of brightness, and has a serene, gay, softly exciting character . . . . Hence in painting it belongs to the illumined and emphatic side." But yellow could be readily "contaminated," which might have disagreeable results: "Thus, the color of sulphur, which inclines to green, has something unpleasant in it . . . . By a slight and scarcely perceptible change, the beautiful impression of fire and gold is transformed into one not undeserving the epithet foul; and the color of honor and joy reversed to that of ignominy and aversion." About carmine red: "The effect of this color is as peculiar as its nature. It conveys an impression of gravity and dignity, and at the same time of grace and attractiveness." In red-yellow energy was high: "The red-yellow gives an impression of warmth and gladness, since it represents the hue of the intenser glow of fire, and the milder radiance of the setting sun . . . . It is not to be wondered at that impetuous, robust, uneducated men, should be especially pleased with this color."

Among the "minus" colors were blue, red-blue (violet), and blue-red (purple). Regarding blue: "This color has a peculiar and almost indescribable effect on the eye. As a hue it is powerful, but it is on the negative side, and in its highest purity, as it were, a stimulating negation. Its appearance, then, is a kind of contradiction between excitement and repose." About violet: "Blue deepens very mildly into red, and then acquires a somewhat active character, although it is on the passive side . . . . It may be said to distract rather than enliven."

Although Goethe disliked yellow-green, he had a fondness for green itself: "If yellow and blue, which we consider as the most fundamental and simple colors, are united as they first appear, in the first state of their action, the color which we call green is the result. The eye experiences a distinctly grateful impression from this color." If the green were perfectly balanced between yellow and blue, "The beholder has neither the wish nor the power to imagine a state beyond it. Hence for rooms to live in constantly, the green color is most generally selected." In terms of harmony yellow and blue were a poor combination. Yellow and red had "a serene and magnificent effect." Orange and purple were exciting and elevating. "The juxtaposition of yellow and green has always something ordinary, but in a cheerful sense; blue and green, on the other hand, is ordinary in a repulsive sense. Our good forefathers called these last fool's colors."

For harmony he favored complements, as did Chevreul later. Referring to a color circle, he wrote that yellow demanded red-blue; blue demanded red-yellow; red demanded green "and contrariwise." He expected artists to have a suitable knowledge of color order and harmony. "A dread, nay, a decided aversion for all theoretical views respecting color and everything belonging to it, has been hitherto found to exist among painters; a prejudice for which, after all, they were not to be blamed; for what has been hitherto called theory was groundless, vacillating, and akin to empiricism." Goethe did his best to remedy this.

EUGÈNE DELACROIX

In his day Delacroix fought for color as against form and became the idol of the impressionists. He was a keen observer of color phenomena in nature and was eager for knowledge. He wrote: "The elements of color theory have been neither analyzed nor taught in our schools of art, because in France it is considered superfluous to study the laws of color, according to the saying, 'Draftsmen may be made, but colorists are born.' Secrets of color theory? Why call those principles secrets which all artists must know and all should have been taught?" Delacroix has been admired and remembered for such incisive comments as, "The enemy of all color is gray . . . . Banish all the earth colors . . . . Give me mud and I will make the skin of a Venus with it, if you will allow me to surround it as I please."

Delacroix had a remarkable vision and curiosity regarding color. Here is a delightful quotation from his *Journal.* "From my window I see a joiner working, naked to the waist, in a gallery. I notice how strongly the half-tones of flesh are colored as compared with inert matter. I noticed the same thing yesterday in the Place Saint Sulpice, where a loafer had climbed up on the statues of the fountain, in the sun. Dull orange in the carnations, the strongest violets for the cast shadows, and golden reflections in the shadows which were relieved against the ground. The orange and violet tints dominated alternately, or mingled. The golden tone had green in it. Flesh only shows its true color in the open air, and above all in the sun. When a man puts his head out of the window he is quite different to what he was inside. Hence the folly of studio studies, which do their best to falsify this color." His criticism of "studio studies," his plea for the observance of colors in the "open air," excited and inspired the young impressionists of his day, some of whom became painters of the outdoors who actually painted out of doors!

M. E. CHEVREUL

Delacroix was an admirer of one M. E. Chevreul, French chemist and head of dyestuffs at the famous Gobelin tapestry works outside Paris. Although at one time Delacroix sought to meet Chevreul, a meeting never took place, due perhaps to the declining health of Chevreul (who lived to be 103). In any event in 1835 Chevreul published one of the greatest books on color ever written, *The Principles of Harmony and Contrast of Colors.* In it were references to "painting, interior decoration, tapestries, carpets, mosaics, colored glazing, paper-staining, calico-printing, letterpress printing, map-coloring, dress, landscape and flower gardening, etc." He was later honored by the French government with a bronze medal, statue, and special edition of his masterwork on the occasion of his hundredth birthday.

Chevreul's creative efforts in the field of color are eminent in three major respects. First, although abstract art did not exist at his time, Chevreul's discussions and graphic illustrations of afterimages and alternate- and simultaneous-contrast effects definitely influenced later nonrepresentational painters and schools of painting such as op art. His findings have subsequently been copied, emulated, and plagiarized. Second, his studies of optical color mixtures influenced impressionism, neoimpressionism, and all forms of color expression involving visual phenomena. Third, he was one of the first men ever to set forth definite principles of color harmony (to be shortly presented), which have been basic to color education and training ever since.

What did Chevreul teach about color harmony? First of all, he differentiated between harmonies of analogy and harmonies of contrast. The latter were his first favorites. "The greater the difference between the colors, the more their association will be favorable to their mutual contrast; and the nearer they are alike, the greater the risk that their association will prove injurious to their beauty." Assuming that the reader has had some training in academic color harmony, let me review what dozens of books have repeated. Consider a conventional color circle such as that used by Chevreul. It has red, yellow, blue primaries; orange, green, violet secondaries; and intermediate hues such as red-orange, yellow-orange, red-violet.

There are harmonies of analogy, colors that lie next to each other on the color circle: red with red-orange, orange, red-violet, or violet. There are harmonies of direct opposites or complements: red with green, yellow with violet, orange with blue, all of which lie opposite each other on the color circle. There are harmonies of split-complements: a base color with the two hues that lie on the sides of its direct complement. Examples would be red with yellow-green and blue-green, yellow with red-violet and blue-violet, blue with red-orange and yellow-orange. There are harmonies of triads, three colors that lie equidistant from each other on the circle, such are red, yellow, blue; orange, green, violet; yellow-orange, blue-green, red-violet. There are harmonies of tetrads, four colors that lie equidistant from each other on the circle, such as red, yellow-orange, green, blue-violet; yellow, blue-green, violet, red-orange; blue, red-violet, orange, yellow-green. Chevreul further noted that "When two colors are bad together, it is always advantageous to separate them by white." Black was also appropriate to separate colors. Gray, however, was "inferior to black and white."

Chevreul's lasting influence on modern forms of art centered around his law of simultaneous contrast. How did it operate? To quote: "If we look simultaneously upon two stripes of different tones of the same color, or upon two stripes of the same tone of different colors placed side by side, if the stripes are not too wide, the eye perceives certain modifications which in the first place influence the intensity of color and in the second, the optical composition of the two juxtaposed colors respectively. All the phenomena I have observed seem to me to depend upon a very simple law, which, taken in its most general significance, may be expressed in these terms: *In the case where the eye sees at the same time two contiguous colors, they will appear as dissimilar as possible, both in their optical composition and in the height of their tone.*" In other words, colors of different *hue* will tend to "spread" still farther apart from each other; colors of different *value* (brightness) will tend to appear still lighter and darker by contrast.

Chevreul then proceeded to give long lists and examples of such contrast. Surprising effects were due both to the influence of afterimages and to the singular results of different colors confused or blended on the retina of the eye. Much of this is academic today, but in Chevreul's time the facts were startling. In case the reader is not too well versed in matters of simultaneous color contrast, here are some examples. If an area of red is seen next to an area of yellow, the afterimage of red (green) will tend to make the yellow appear greenish. The violet afterimage of the yellow will similarly make the red appear purplish. Complements, however, enhance and lend brilliance to each other. If red and green are juxtaposed, both will have heightened power because of their afterimages. As Chevreul wrote: "Red, the complementary of green, added to red, increases its intensity. Green, the complementary of red, added to green, augments its intensity."

On the problem of optical mixtures (fine lines or small dots of a color mixed on the retina of the eye) Chevreul was able to draw upon a wealth of color experience gained in the making of Gobelin and Beauvais tapestries and Savonnerie carpets, French textiles of world eminence. His conclusions were that "there is a *mixture of colors* whenever materials of various colors are so divided and then combined that the eye cannot distinguish these materials from each other; in which case the eye receives a single impression." This impression differed from that of colors seen in large areas side by side. The American Ogden Rood would later prove to be more perceptive in the matter of visual color mixtures.

OGDEN N. ROOD

Ogden N. Rood of Columbia University in New York became America's leading authority on physiological optics upon the publication in 1879 of his book *Modern Chromatics*, which in later editions had the title *Students' Text-Book of Color*. Although a scientist by training, Rood had considerable talent as an artist and hence could well interpret technical data in terms of intelligible aesthetics. What is remarkable about Rood is that his book, translated into French in 1881, became the bible of the neoimpressionists and was avidly read by such painters as Camille Pissarro, Georges Seurat, and Paul Signac.

Rood had written: "We refer to the custom of placing a quantity of small dots of two colors very near each other, and allowing them to be blended by the eye at the proper distance. . . . The results obtained in this way are true mixtures of colored light. . . . This method is almost the only practical one at the disposal of the artist whereby he can actually mix, not pigments, but masses of colored light." Here was the principle of the divisionist technique that was studied (but for shorter periods) by other painters such as Van Gogh, Henri Matisse, Emil Bernard, Toulouse-Lautrec. Unique examples of divisionism by these artists have survived.

Rood advised Albert H. Munsell on the development of Munsell's color sphere. Because of his skill in art his book had chapters on painting, decoration, and harmony. He granted that form was more important than color in realistic painting, but "In decorative art the element of color is more important than form." He repeated many of the experiments of Chevreul and spoke of the harmony of opposites, adjacents, triads. He presented extensive lists of bad, inferior, disagreeable, tolerable, and excellent color combinations. Like Goethe, he felt that "green and blue, for example, make a poor combination, and yet it is one constantly occurring in nature, as in the case where the blue sky is seen through green foliage." Munsell perhaps borrowed from Rood in the following statement from *Modern Chromatics*: "We return now to the proposition that the best effect is produced when the colors in a design are present in such proportions that a composite mixture of them would produce a neutral gray."

Rood brought credit to America. His masterwork has been justly reprinted in recent times (1973). He stood for knowledge, discipline—and talent—as requisites in art.

WASSILY KANDINSKY

Few painters have been great color theorists. Da Vinci is one exception. Sir Joshua Reynolds was essentially a lecturer rather than a teacher. Delacroix, though a shrewd observer of nature, did not attempt to formalize or organize his many keen observations on color. In modern art, however, the name of Wassily Kandinsky holds a romantic if not exalted place. Among color theorists he has developed one of the most fanciful and esoteric of theories. His ideas have been carried out on his own canvases. He has exploited the spectrum to produce some of the rarest abstractions in the craft of painting—effects in which form is definitely second to color.

Kandinsky, like most painters, was an individualist. Personality tinged all his postulations. To him colors had a psychic effect just as they had a physical quality. "They produce a corresponding spiritual vibration, and it is only as a step towards this spiritual vibration that the elementary physical impression is of importance." This meant that color had strange powers and that the problems of harmony must contemplate the spirit of man as well as his vision. "It is evident . . . that color harmony must rest only on a corresponding vibration in the human soul; and this is one of the guiding principles of the inner need."

The spectrum had major dimensions of warmth and coldness, lightness and darkness. Thus colors could have four shades of appeal—warm and light or warm and dark, cold and light or cold and dark. Blue and yellow were dominant. "Generally speaking, warmth or cold in a color means an approach respectively to yellow or to blue." Movement was to be found among primary colors. Yellow had a maximum spreading action. It was inclined to white and tended to approach the observer. Blue was inclined to black, moved in upon itself, and retreated. "The power of profound meaning is blue."

"Red rings inwardly with a determined and powerful intensity. It glows in itself, maturely, and does not distribute its vigor aimlessly."

"Orange is red brought nearer to humanity by yellow."

"Violet is red withdrawn from humanity by blue."

It was Kandinsky's belief that "keen" colors (yellow) were best suited to sharp forms, and soft, deep colors (blue) to round forms. Shape also affected appeal. The same hue could be given different spiritual values through different forms.

ALBERT H. MUNSELL

Albert H. Munsell is the most famous of American colorists. His Color Sphere, developed at the turn of the century, has since been improved upon by American scientists and is the most widely used system of color notation in existence today. A text of his, *A Color Notation,* originally published in 1905, has been kept in print ever since. My editing of Munsell's theories of color harmony (not the technical aspects of his color solid) has been devoted to *A Grammar of Color*, written by T. M. Cleland in 1921 but with brief chapters contributed by Munsell himself before he died in 1918.

Munsell in his day had the conservative taste of late Victorians. There are amusing quotations that voice his opinions. "The sense of comfort is the outcome of balance, while marked unbalance immediately urges a corrective." This required restraint. "The use of strongest colors only fatigues the eyes, which is also true of the weakest colors." The French school of fauvism would dispute this conservatism, as would most modern artists. "Beginners should avoid strong color," while "Quiet color is a mark of good taste."

"The circus wagon and poster, although they yell successfully for momentary attention, soon become so painful to the vision that one turns from them." Finally, "If we wish our children to become well-bred, is it logical to begin by encouraging barbarous tastes?"

Munsell's principles of harmony, to be now reviewed, are taught in many schools today. They tend to be strict and academic, to confine expression rather than set it free. In the Cleland book mentioned above I have described (and illustrated in full color) nine of Munsell's principles, which are given here.

1. Munsell makes a prominent feature of colors that have medium value (brightness) and medium chroma (a term he devised), or purity. With a scale of nine gray steps, a combination of steps 1 (black), 5 (medium gray), 9 (white) would be ideal. So would steps 3, 5, 7 and 4, 5, 6, with 5 always a point of balance. Light accents on dark or dark accents on light would be appropriate but with value 5 as a fulcrum.

2. Monochromatic harmonies involving one key hue should also follow the above principle. Ideal would be a color of medium 5 value and medium 5 chroma combined (a) with a 3 or 7 or 4 or 6 value of the same hue or (b) with 3 or 7 or 2 or 8 chromas. Diagonal monochromatic harmonies could also be arranged but again with 5/5 as the key.

3. As with Chevreul, complementary colors were quite harmonious but with special reservations. Once again, a red of 5 value could be com-

bined harmoniously with a blue-green of 5 value on a value-5 gray. Or a chroma-5 red could be combined with a chroma-5 blue-green on a value-5 gray. Other complements would, of course, be equally concordant.

4. Quite individual to Munsell was the contention that 5 balance was desirable. In this principle a red of 3 chroma, for example, would need a blue-green of 3 chroma to balance. But if the red had a 6 chroma, a blue-green area twice the size would be necessary for balance.

5. As with principle 4, if different values were involved, any stronger chroma should occupy less area than a weaker chroma. *Beauty could be proved if all areas were measured and put on a disk, and if the spun result was a neutral value-5 gray, all would be well!*

6. Different chromas and different values could be neatly arranged as in principle 5 but with the measured result ever passing through the magic value 5.

7. Neighboring hues could be combined with split-complements but balanced as above.

8. Diminishing sequences from light to dark values and from pure to weak chromas could be plotted throughout the solid.

9. Elliptical paths could be arranged—complicated but beautiful.

These principles of Munsell may lead to harmony, but unfortunately most of them tend to result in muted and grayed combinations that hardly reflect the modern taste and preference for bright hues.

WILHELM OSTWALD

If color solids and color systems are to be considered for purposes of harmony, the principles of Ostwald are superior to those of Munsell. (I have given elaborate attention to both systems.) With Ostwald there is less emphasis on value and chroma and more on qualities of whiteness and/or blackness in color.

Unlike Rood and Munsell, both of whom were practicing artists, Wilhelm Ostwald was a scientist who won the Nobel Prize for chemistry in 1909. He took an interest in the problems of color organization, created an original concept of color order (with due tribute to Ewald Hering, a German psychologist), and gained worldwide fame as an authority on color. A text of his, *Die Farbenfibel,* was published in 1916 and ran into 15 editions. In a recent English translation, *The Color Primer* (1969), this writer has added a chapter on the history of color systems and has appended an evaluation of Ostwald's achievements.

Whereas Munsell placed emphasis on value and chroma, Ostwald dealt with qualities of whiteness and blackness in color. A rational form for color was the triangle, with pure hue (C) on one angle, white (W) on the second, and black (B) on the third. All possible variations of a given hue could be plotted within this triangle: $C + W + B = 1$.

Ostwald's theories of harmony can be simply stated. Any colors that have the same hue, white, and black content will be harmonious (regardless of value differences). Color scales parallel to CW have equal black content, and with such scales the deeper tone will be pure and the lighter tone weak. Color scales parallel to CB have equal white content, and with them the lighter tone will be pure and the deeper tone dull. Color scales parallel to WB (vertical scales) were great favorites of Ostwald. He called them the "shadow series" and likened them to the chiaroscuro modeling of the Renaissance painters. These scales had an apparent equal-hue content. More complex were "ring-star" harmonies, which, like the diminishing sequences and elliptical paths of Munsell, plotted concordant steps within the color solid but with careful respect for balance of white, black, or hue content.

Maitland Graves has written a good book on Munsell. One of the best on Ostwald is by Egbert Jacobson (see the Bibliography). Other recommended books that include notes on harmony will be found in Johannes Itten, Josef Albers, Paul Klee, Frans Garritsen. For other principles of color harmony, less academic than those discussed herewith, consult my own books, most of which seek to create new modes of color expression drawn from the wonders and phenomena of human perception.

COLOR PREFERENCES

Dozens of color-preference tests (color for the sake of color) have been conducted over the years. With infants, for example, who no doubt are influenced more by visual attraction than by emotional pleasure, luminous colors such as yellow, white, pink, red will be stared at longest. In children a liking for yellow begins to drop away—and to keep dropping with the years. Their preference is then for red and blue, universal favorites, which maintain their fascination throughout life. With maturity comes a greater liking for hues of shorter wavelength (blue, green) than for hues of longer wavelength (red, orange, yellow). The order now becomes blue, red, green, violet, orange, yellow. And it remains thus, the eternal and international ranking.

That color preferences are almost identical in human beings of both sexes and in persons of all nationalities and creeds is substantiated on every side. T. R. Garth found that American Indians preferred red, blue, violet, green, orange, yellow. Among Filipinos the order was red, green, blue, violet, orange, yellow. Among Negroes the order was blue, red, green, violet, orange, yellow—the same as for practically everybody else. Even among insane subjects S. E. Katz found almost the same rankings—blue, green, red, violet, yellow, orange. Green was best liked by male inmates, and red by female. Warm hues seemed to appeal to morbid patients, and cool hues to the more hysterical ones.

To summarize the whole picture, H. J. Eysenck tabulated a mass of research involving some 21,060 individual judgments. Blue ranked first, then red, green, violet, orange, and yellow. In a similar recapitulation of sex differences the order was the same except that, while men put orange in fifth place and yellow in sixth, women put yellow in fifth place and orange in sixth.

COLOR COMBINATIONS

A great deal of research has also been devoted to color combinations. In working with children M. Imada found that color preference was not haphazard even though good discrimination was not highly developed. Given black crayons, the youngsters were inclined to draw inanimate things—vehicles, buildings. When the same children were given colored crayons, their fancies were more inspired to attempt human beings, animals, and plants. Red with yellow and red with blue were favored combinations. In similar experiments Ann Van Nice Gale found yellow popular in combination with red-violet or blue. The combination of blue and green was also liked. Contrast, naturally, was more exciting than analogy or subtlety.

Using colored lights thrown upon a screen, William E. Walton and Beulah M. Morrison found the combination of red and blue highest in rank with adults, then blue and green, red and green, clear and blue, amber and blue, amber and green, red and amber, and clear and amber. More on the color preferences of children and adults and their meaning in terms of personality is found in Chapter IX.

J. P. GUILFORD

J. P. Guilford has conducted a number of technical queries on the harmony of color combinations. He believes that more is involved here than mere emotional pleasure. "I think that it is more than a figure of speech to say that living tissue, particularly brain tissue, generates colors and pleasantness or unpleasantness just as other collections of matter generate the phenomenon of heat, or magnetism, or electricity."

Concerning harmonious arrangements he writes: "There is some evidence that either very small or very large differences in hue give more pleasing results than do medium differences. This tendency is much stronger for women than for men." Thus a person is likely to see harmony either in colors that are closely related or in those that are antithetical and opposite—not in other relationships. To visualize a color circle, yellow, for example, will seem harmonious with yellow-orange and yellow-green; blue with blue-violet or violet. It will not be particularly well liked in combination with orange, green, or even red. Guilford has likewise determined through research that, if the choice is between grayish tones and pure hues, the pure forms will be preferred. If the choice is between dark tones and light tones, the light tones will be preferred.

There are relationships of color with music, food, odors, shapes and forms, tactile qualities of warmth and coolness, and moods. More information is found in my *Color Psychology and Color Therapy* and also in other chapters of this book.

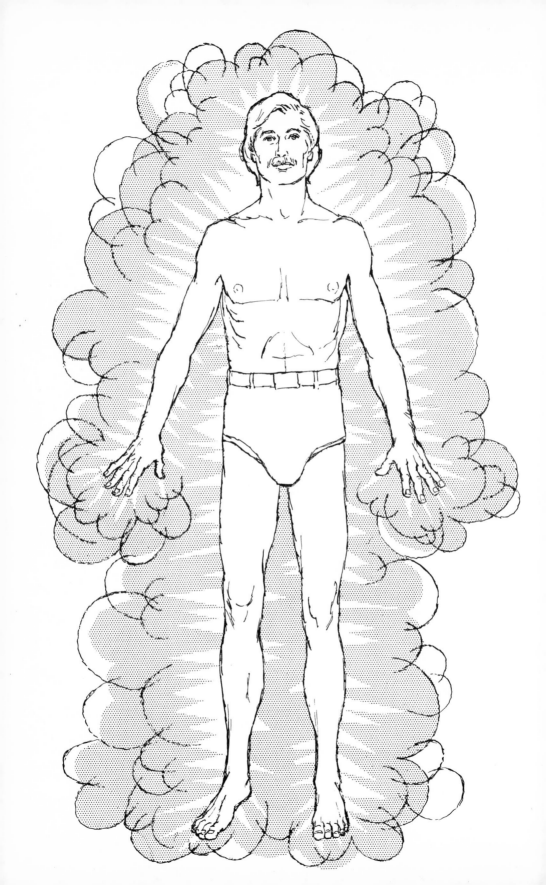

VI. Psychic Response

This chapter is concerned with emanations, visible and invisible, with auras, the astral body, corona discharge, bioplasma body, and with modern terms such as electrodynamics, psychotronics, and biodynamics, which have in recent years become matters of serious scientific investigation and popular exploitation.

As a writer on the field of color, I am often criticized for my interest in the occult and attitude toward things psychic and mystical. Many of my censors are insistent on *facts*, which I all too often cannot submit. This does not bother me unduly. The world is full of mysteries that have no patent explanation, particularly concerning phenomena associated with the psychological. In my defense let me call upon the great Albert Einstein, who admitted, "I didn't arrive at my understanding of the fundamental laws of the universe through my rational mind." Thomas Edison worked on apparatus to communicate with the dead. Freud was intrigued by psychic phenomena (dreams!) and wrote papers on telepathy and the occult. Jung was concerned with skin responses and wrote that "the skin's electrical activity changed remarkably when [a person's] ears heard words associated with emotion." I admire the conclusion of B. W. Kouwer in his *Colors and their Character:* "Phenomenology does not posit any facts at all . . . [it] deals with color only *in so far* as it is experienced, and not as a physical fact or abstract concept; it deals with the observer only *in so far* as he experiences the color, and not as a physiological mechanism."

A man's interest in the occult by no means reflects on other of his convictions. Arguments can be presented both to prove and to disprove the existence of gods. What is significant to my mind is man's fascination with that which surpasses his understanding. So it is with me. Why do millions of human beings believe in supernatural powers, in astrology; why are they superstitious, credulous, gullible about enigmas that make little or no sense in factual terms?

THE ANCIENT AND THE MODERN MYSTIC

In the mystic approach nearly all early civilizations used color as a token of the loftier qualities of human culture. There were certain philosophers, however, who went beyond the formal symbolism of the mysteries and studied the auric light that was thought to issue from the body. Here the true marks of culture were to be found, as unmistakable as the rainbow, visible, actual, and the real index to a man's inherent qualities, good and bad.

Man had been likened to a celestial body that emits vibrations of light. This concept usually referred to the sun or to a supreme invisible deity whose rays gave life and spirit to humans. The halos, robes, insignias, jewels, and ornaments used on their own persons and on the effigies of their gods symbolized the spiritual energies that radiated from the body. The elaborate headdress of the Egyptian and the nimbus of the Christian saint represented the auric bodies of the elect. These streams were supposed to pour from the surface of the flesh, and their colors were a gauge of cultural development, spiritual perfection, and physical health.

To the mystic all plants and animals emitted an aura. (This has been confirmed in modern times.) In man the aura was as much a part of his entity as his body. Celebrated men such as Benvenuto Cellini had noted it: "Ever since the time of my strange vision until now an aureole of glory (marvelous to relate) has rested on my head. This is visible to every sort of men to whom I have chosen to point it out; but there have been very few. This halo can be observed above my shadow in the morning from the rising of the sun for about two hours, and far better when the grass is drenched with dew."

Edwin D. Babbitt in his celebrated book *The Principles of Light and Color* presented a good deal of material on the work of Mrs. Minnie Weston concerning the psychic colors that are said to issue from the brain. These hues comprised what Babbitt termed the "odic atmosphere." He pointed out first of all a need for harmony between the vibrations of the world and the human body and recommended that a person should sleep with his head to the north to "lie in the magnetic meridian." (The worst position was with the head to the west.) Odic light appeared in various forms—as incandescence; as flame; as threads, streaks, or nebulas; as smoke; and as sparks. The odic atmosphere was thought to be twice as fine as ordinary atmosphere because its vibrations were supposed to be twice as fine as those of light.

The trance medium Edgar Cayce recently declared that he saw color surrounding most persons. These interpretations of his, however, were conventionally those of the mystic. Red was for force, vigor, and energy; orange was for thoughtfulness and consideration; yellow, for health and wellbeing; green was the color of healing; blue was the color of the spirit; indigo and violet indicated those searching for religious experience. Like his predecessors, he wrote: "The perfect color, of course, is white, and this is what we are all striving for. If our souls were in perfect balance, then all our color vibrations would blend and we would have an aura of pure white." Edgar Cayce foresaw great practical value in the study of the aura. It could be interpreted for purposes of diagnosis and therapy—and this will be seen in the pages that follow. He cautioned, "But I do not think that color therapy will become widespread or practical until we have accepted the truth of auras and become accustomed to reading them in order to discover what unbalance is disturbing a person."

THE CLINICAL APPROACH

In color is a psychic factor, appealing, emotional, in every way inspiring and suggestive of mysterious powers. Before discussing what modern medicine is willing to admit about color and the aura let me shift from the occult viewpoint to the clinical. The study of the human aura and of astral light is not always a matter of mysticism and abracadabra. Even the most incredulous person is forced to admit that emanations of some sort issue from the human body. This can not only be sensed as heat or odor, but under proper conditions it can actually be seen. Sir Oliver Lodge, who was attracted to spiritual phenomena, wrote, "All evidence tends to convince me that we have an Etheric body as well as a physical body . . . it is the organized entity that builds up the body."

THE GREAT FRANZ MESMER

A bridge from the astral emanations of the mystic to the energy fields recognized by the modern scientist was crossed in principle as far back as the seventeenth century. In 1679 one William Maxwell wrote a treatise, *De Medicina Magnetica*, in which he stated the following: "Material rays flow from all bodies in which the soul operates by its presence. By these rays energy and the power of working are diffused. The vital spirit which descends from the sky, pure, unchanged, and whole, is the parent of the vital spirit which exists in all things. If you make use of the universal spirit by means of instruments impregnated with this spirit you will thereby call to your aid the great secret of the ages. The universal medicine is nothing but the vital spirit repeated in the proper subject."

This grand assumption later inspired the great father of hypnotism, Franz Anton Mesmer (1733?–1815). He became an expert in animal magnetism, studied in Vienna, and opened a famous clinic in Paris that drew patients from all of Europe. Mesmer declared, "A mutual influence subsists between the celestial bodies, the earth, and living bodies." He devised a magnetic oval tub that was surrounded by chairs or benches on which the patients sat. The contrivance was described at the time in these words: "M. Mesmer, Doctor of Medicine of the Faculty of Vienna, in Austria, is the sole discoverer of animal magnetism. This method of curing a multitude of ailments—hydropsy, paralysis, gout, scurvy, blindness, and accidental deafness among others—consists in the application of a fluid or agent which M. Mesmer directs upon those who resort to him, sometimes with one of his fingers and sometimes with an iron rod held by another and pointed as he chooses. He also employs a tub furnished with attached cords, which the sick persons tie round themselves, and with bent-iron bars, which they approach to the pit of their stomach, their liver, or their spleen, or, in general, to any part of their body in which they suffer. The sick persons, especially the females, go into convulsions or fits which bring about their cure. The Magnetizers [they are those to whom M. Mesmer has revealed his secret, and are more than a hundred in number, among them counting the first nobles of the court] place their hands upon the part affected and rub it for some time; this operation hastens the effect of the cords and irons. Every other day there is a tub for the poor; in the antechamber musicians play airs calculated to induce gaiety in the sick persons. Men and women of every age and every degree are seen arriving in crowds at this celebrated physician's house—the soldier with his badges of honour, the lawyer, the monk, the man of letters, the blue-ribbon cook, the artisan, the physician, the surgeon. It is a spectacle truly worthy of feeling souls to see men distinguished by birth or social rank magnetizing, with tender solicitude, children, aged persons, and, above all, the necessitous. As for M. Mesmer, he breathes an air of beneficence in all his discourse; he is grave and speaks little. His head seems always filled with great thoughts." Mesmer's clientele was quite eminent. He could also magnetize water and use it as a therapeutic elixir. Though he was praised by some, others looked upon his work as that of the devil. Thus he was a great benefactor and a charlatan at one and the same time.

GEORGE STARR WHITE

In modern times a number of investigators have studied the auric scene. Let me refer to the work of George Starr White, Walter J. Kilner, and Oscar Bagnall.

The Story of the Human Aura, written by George Starr White, took a fairly middle course between the eloquent viewpoint of the mystic and the modest viewpoint of the scientist. Agreeing with Mesmer, White declared that a magnetic atmosphere surrounded animals and plants. These emanations differed and were subject to change. By accepting them one may account for the mysteries of thought transference, the weird prescience of strange happenings that often strikes a person. He stated that health and disease made themselves evident in the aura. And the rays changed in appearance when a person turned towards different points of the compass. "No matter what form life or vital force may take, no matter what vehicle life is carried in—be it animate or inanimate—its magnetic atmosphere must be characteristic of the vehicle." White concluded that the magnetic emanations from the forefinger of the left hand and the thumb of the right hand were positive and that the emanations from the forefinger of the right hand and the thumb of the left hand were negative. He described an auric cabinet to study the phenomenon. The color of the average aura was grayish blue. (Kirlian photography, discussed later in this chapter, has now been used to take actual photographs of auras.)

WALTER J. KILNER

A more logical and unprejudiced attitude is found in Walter J. Kilner's book *The Human Atmosphere.* Kilner very deliberately shunned the mystic aspects of auric light and made his investigation with all the sedulity of a laboratory worker. His conclusions: surrounding the human body is a visible envelope that consists of three definite parts. First is a narrow, dark band a quarter of an inch wide, which is adjacent to the skin. Beyond this and projecting from two to four inches outward is a second aura. This is the clearest of all. And beyond this is a third aura, misty in aspect and without sharp outline on its farther edge. This is generally about six inches across. The radiations normally shoot out at right angles from the body. These inner rays are electric in appearance and have a fugitive quality, shifting and changing. Longer rays project from the fingers, the elbows, knees, hips, and breasts. The color of health is a bluish gray, according to Kilner, tinged with yellow and red. A grayer and duller color is typical of a diseased body. Kilner, however, preferred to base his diagnoses on the shape of the aura rather than on its chromatic qualities.

OSCAR BAGNALL

Kilner's work was taken up and vastly improved by Oscar Bagnall. In *The Origin and Properties of the Human Aura* a number of engaging theories are set forth, as well as a detailed explanation of the procedure to follow in making the aura visible. Some may observe it merely by gazing at a person in a dimly illuminated room. Bagnall, however, following the example of Kilner, makes use of a special screen.

He divides the aura into two parts, an inner and an outer. The inner aura, about three inches across, is marked by a clear brightness and rays that shoot out in straight lines. This aura is approximately the same in all persons. It may also be supplemented by special bundles of rays emanating from various parts of the body that are not necessarily parallel to the other rays. The outer aura, which is more filmy, enlarges with age and generally has greater dimension in women than in men. Its average width is about six inches. Color is best seen here—bluish or grayish. The bluer the hue, the finer the intellect; the grayer the tone, the duller the intellect. The outer aura is subject to radical change due to mood or disease. Bagnall declares that no aura shines from any dead thing.

In studying the aura the eye is first sensitized by gazing at the sky through a special dicyanin (blue) filter. The observer then sits with his back to the window. A feeble illumination is permitted to enter the room. The patient, naked, stands before a neutral screen. According to Bagnall, auric light has definite wavelengths that lie beyond the visible spectrum. Because blue and violet rays are seen better by the rods of the eye than by the cones, the blue filter tends to eliminate the longer red and orange rays of light and to emphasize the violet. The sensitizing of the eye can also be achieved by first gazing at areas of yellow paper, which fatigue the retinal nerves to red and green and at the same time bring out a stronger response to blue.

According to Bagnall, organic diseases seem to affect the inner aura. The emanating rays may lose their sparkle and appear dull or limpid. Intellectual and nervous disorders, puberty, and menstruation seem to affect the outer aura. With disease certain dark patches may appear. More telling, however, is the general shape of the aura. An aura that falls away suddenly in the neighborhood of the thigh may indicate that a person suffers from a nervous complaint. An outward bulge away from the spine is a typical sign of hysteria. Neurotics usually have a poor outer aura and a dull inner aura. Physical disturbances seem to affect brightness. Nervous conditions seem to affect the quality of hue. Bagnall diagnoses pregnancy as follows: The aura becomes broader and deeper over the breasts. There is a widening of the haze in the area immediately below the navel. There is a slight decrease in the clearness of the bluish color, a phenomenon that changes as pregnancy advances. He feels that medicine and surgery may be served through further clinical study. These emanations that stream from the body apparently have profound significance. This view and assumption have been well supported and verified in recent times, as is discussed below.

THE HUMAN AURA

The human aura is one realm in which the mystics of old have won striking victories in modern times. What many skeptics once looked upon as abstruse conjecture now turns out to be definite fact. Auras were seen and believed in centuries before electromagnetic energy was known to exist. Anyone today who doubts the reality of human emanations (over and above heat, odor, and moisture) himself dwells in the limbo of the past. The human body transmits a series of electronic or magnetic fields. Their emissions can be measured with modern equipment such as the electroencephalograph (EEG), which measures brain waves. Energy comes forth from all organs of the body and from the skin itself. The old mystic and the modern scientist are brought together in the same laboratory.

KIRLIAN PHOTOGRAPHY

Let me begin with what is known as Kirlian photography. (If the reader is knowledgeable in this area, please forgive this summary.) Articles and books are written today about "skin talk," in which the body's electrical activity communicates information about personal thoughts and feelings. Kirlian photography photographs auras—and biofeedback techniques reveal emotional and physiological responses to color.

While the mystics spoke of color in glowing and imaginative terms and while other more sober men wrote of rather obscure procedures, Semyon D. and Valentina Kirlian of Russia around 1958 described a method of using high-voltage discharges to photograph "flare patterns" of animate and inanimate things. Fairly successful attempts had been made before, and equally successful attempts have been made since. In what is today known as Kirlian photography the aura has become a matter of tangible and visible record. The world now enters an age of electrodynamics and biodynamics. (A good source of reference here is *The Kirlian Aura* by Stanley Krippner and Daniel Rubin.)

What is seen? To quote Ostrander and Schroeder: "It should be noted that when photographing on multilayer color film with disc plates, different parts of a living man's skin are transposed into different colors. For example, the heart region is intensive blue, the forearm is greenish blue, and the thigh is olive. . . . There is reason to assume that during unexpected emotional experiences (e.g., fear and illness) the inherent color in a section changes. It seems to us that these characteristic appearances merit serious study for diagnostic value in medicine for early detection of a disease. . . . Let us stop to consider several electrical occurrences observed on the skin of a living man. In the visual field, on a background of the configuration of the skin, discharge channels with varying characteristics are visible: point, corona, and flares in the form of luminescent clusters. These are of different colors: blue, lavender, and yellow. They may be bright or faded, constant or of varying intensity, periodically flaring up or constantly flaring, motionless or moving. . . . On some sections of skin, points of blue and gold abruptly flare up. Their characteristic feature is a rhythm of flashes and immobility. . . . The color of the clusters may be milky blue, pale lilac, gray, or orange."

Methods of producing Kirlian or radiation-field photographs are elaborately described in *The Living Aura* by Kendall Johnson. Ostrander and Schroeder in *Handbook of Psi Discoveries* also describe Kirlian techniques and methods in elaborate detail. Through high-voltage discharges—but without lens or camera as such—photographic prints of emissions are recorded. It may not be necessary to describe techniques or equipment, for Kirlian Electrophotographic Units are now on the market (1976) through the Edmund Scientific Company of New Jersey. Through electrophotographs of the finger Johnson reached a number of interesting conclusions. "Rest, relaxation, feeling at ease seemed to be correlated with a wide, bright, smooth corona. . . . Fear or apprehension tended to produce a weak, interrupted corona with a blotch."

Kirlian or radiation-field photographs have yet to be made of the body at large. The human aura from head to foot, described by the mystics of old and by Kilner and Bagnall in more modern times, has yet to be recorded on any huge photographic film or plate. This may not be necessary, for through the study of brain waves and skin responses with excellent equipment much is learned of man's physical and emotional constitution.

DIAGNOSTIC REVELATIONS

To continue with the aura, there are clear indications that shifts and changes may indicate and actually anticipate physiological and psychological conditions in an individual. In psychosomatic medicine, in which environmental conditions may lead to tension, fear, depression and in which these in turn may lead to a number of physiological ailments, a study of the aura may be of great aid in diagnosis. Emotional states can be detected in various ways: with the electroencephalograph (which records brain waves) as well as through hormone production, pupil dilation, finger pressure, palmar conductance.

The very existence of the aura may help to explain or at least to confirm psychic healing, in which certain rare persons can through "the laying on of hands" offer relief in some conditions of human distress. There are some recognized researchers who believe that through Kirlian photography there is visible evidence of a flow of energy, or interaction, between human beings and their environments and that with psychic healers the corona of the healer may flow into the being of the person being treated. This may seem farfetched, but liberal psychosomatic medicine does not totally reject any such "miracles." Thelma Moss, in her splendid book *The Probability of the Impossible*, offers a good description of Kirlian photography. On the matter of healing she writes, "I do believe that the pictures [Kirlian] show that the energy can travel not only from healer to patient, but from patient to healer." There is also a flow of energy or interaction between persons and their environment. A healer with a wide corona may transmit energy to a person with a narrow corona. Incidentally, there are forty references to spiritual healing in the Bible.

ACUPUNCTURE

Electronic devices have been developed to locate acupuncture (hoku) points in the human body. The Russians have the tobiscope, and Kendall Johnson describes one of his own invention. The Russian tobiscope lights up when acupuncture points are touched and is thus a useful device for the acupuncture specialist. Whether or not acupuncture is embraced or rejected by the medical profession, one must not forget that the Chinese have recognized it for a few thousand years. Eisenhower's physician, Paul Dudley White, who visited China, wisely wrote: "If it were useless, it would have been dropped thousands of years ago. There's something in it, but it's difficult to say just what." Could it be that acupuncture needs faith and mysticism to support it?

BIOPLASMIC ENERGY

Corona emanations of the aura may not be traceable wholly to skin temperature, galvanic skin response, electrical or magnetic fields, or perspiration. There may well be other energy involved, phenomena that are unpredicted and unexplained by physical theory. Call it bioplasmic energy or any other term, science no doubt has further and mysterious emanations to comprehend and record.

If the emanations are magnetic, Harold Saxon Burr of Yale maintains, electromagnetic fields within the body are influenced by greater fields throughout the universe—thus confirming the mystic's concept of the little microcosm within the great macrocosm. Burr's unique work is described by Edward W. Russell in *Design for Destiny*. "All living forms—whether they be the human body, animals, trees, plants or lower forms of life—possess, and are controlled, by electromagnetic fields." Emanations may well account for the mysteries of extrasensory perception. "Without benefit of science, thought-transmission has been an *experimentally-proven fact* to countless people since the beginning of man's history. It is an accepted commonplace among husbands and wives, parents and children and others who are mutually-sympathetic."

In his article "Magnetic Fields of the Human Body" David Cohen refers to Mesmer and describes today's methods of checking human magnetic fields. "The body's fields have now been measured in at least ten laboratories, and are the subject of eight doctoral theses and about fifty published papers." The human body is indeed "a source of magnetic fields," and they have been recorded in specially shielded rooms at the Massachusetts Institute of Technology. Cohen remarks that the measurements obtained "of the heart, the brain and the lungs are potentially of value in clinical diagnosis and physiological research."

Psychiatry and Mysticism (edited by Stanley R. Dean) contains excellent chapters by Shafica Karagulla of the Royal College of Physicians in Edinburgh and John C. Pierrakos, a practicing psychiatrist and director of the Institute of Bioenergetic Analysis in New York. Dr. Karagulla describes the three auric fields. The first is the vital energy field. This extends about three to five centimeters beyond the body and has a bluish haze. The second field, which has a changing pattern of colors, reveals a person's emotions. The third field is the mental one, which "exhibits the quality of the mind and thinking of the individual." There is a fourth integrating field. These fields can be used for diagnostic purposes, according to Dr. Karagulla. The energy vortex at the throat has a pale blue or violet color in a healthy person. Red or orange reveals problems in the thyroid that might be detected in advance.

Some gifted doctors have been known to see auras in their patients and to diagnose from them, usually without making any reference whatsoever to the insight. Some psychiatrists declare that mentally disturbed persons may also have a unique odor. Dr. Pierrakos describes the aura and equipment used to measure it. He speaks of three layers or fields. "The principal movement of the three layers can be described as a wave moving away from the body. . . . I consider the field to be primarily an expression of all aspects of man—physical, emotional, mental, and spiritual." These are statements of a psychiatrist, not a mystic! He further wrote: "Human beings seem to swim in a sea of fluid, tinged rhythmically with brilliant colors which constantly change hues, shimmer, and vibrate. In truth, to be alive is to be colorful and vibrant." He noted various changes in illness. Fear caused a dulling effect. Schizophrenic patients showed severe disturbances.

THE SKIN TALKS

Numerous articles and at least one book have been written about "skin talk." (The book is *Touching: The Human Significance of the Skin* by Ashley Montagu.) Virtually everyone has experienced blushing, clammy hands, wet armpits. With the lie detector (polygraph) skin conductance is readily noted and charted. What happens is that electrical impulses are recorded that surprisingly give away a person's feelings—not invariably but generally. The machine can communicate information about a person's emotions. Jung experimented with it and noted that the skin's electrical activity could even be affected by word associations.

"The skin sees in technicolor," writes Barbara B. Brown in her remarkable book *New Mind, New Body*—it can discriminate among colors. "The skin also is a good color detector and seems to reflect the way in which brain neurons process color information. Experiments demonstrating body reactions to color support the common belief that colors induce emotional states which are specific to different hues." When different colors were projected on a screen the polygraph showed stronger response to red than to green—and greater response to violet than to green. The information recorded evidently was picked up by the brain through the eye and then expressed electrically by the skin. Auras obviously are involved here.

BRAIN WAVES

Robert Ornstein and Roger Sperry have developed a theory that the two hemispheres of the brain have different functions. Both men have been concerned with biofeedback techniques and with brain-wave responses. In brief, the left hemisphere of the brain is good at logic, while the right hemisphere is more intuitive. Lawyers were likely to have more active left hemispheres, while artists had more active right hemispheres.

From the polygraph, which measures skin response, to the electro-encephalograph (EEG), which measures brain waves, the aura still shines. Just about all parts of the human body generate electrical current. This is especially true of the brain. If properly amplified, enough electrical energy can be developed to turn lights off and on (and run toy electric trains). So-called biofeedback is developing great popular appeal. There is a Bio-Feedback Research Society, and hundreds of researchers and research reports have been devoted to the phenomenon. The Edmund Scientific Company, which previously was mentioned as the manufacturer of Kirlian photographic equipment, also has available biofeedback monitors and alpha-wave sensors (1976). What was once a scientific development has unfortunately become a pseudoscientific plaything. A GSR Monitor is also made to check the reactions of plants to light, touch, music, the human voice, and smoke.

Through the control of alpha (and other) waves by an individual body reactions can be regulated from the inside out, so to speak. Control of alpha waves as an aid to meditation is showing promise in psychosomatic medicine in the relief of such problems as high blood pressure, migraine headache, insomnia, asthma, and drug rehabilitation. It can also cope with psychological fears, tensions, and frustrations.

As to color, Barbara Brown tried to determine "Whether feelings about color modify brain waves or whether brain waves are first affected by colors and the feelings developed later." Brain-wave activity was recorded when different colors were exposed. She concluded that "The

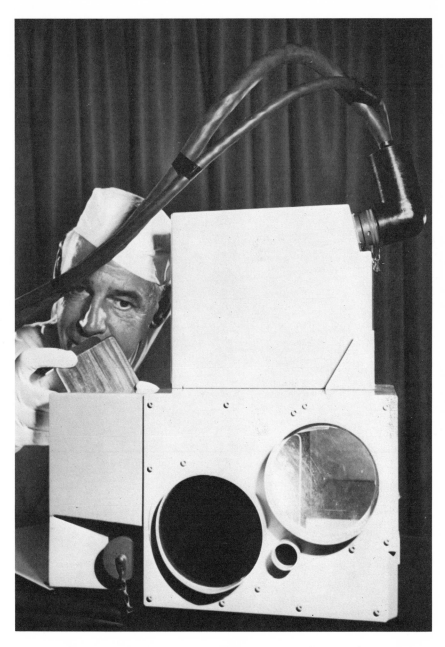

Laser is used as an altimeter in space flight. Coupled with a metric camera, detail views of the lunar surface can be mapped by astronauts. United Press International Photo (see Chapter II).

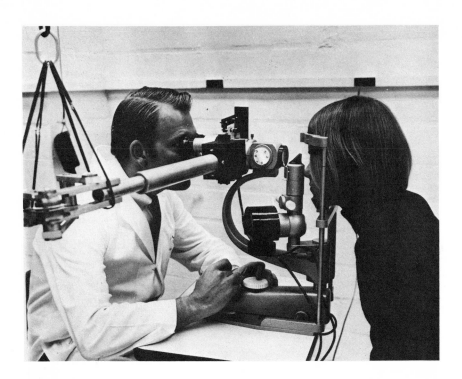

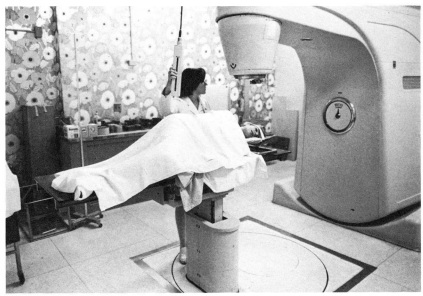

The top illustration shows the use of laser beams for the treatment of eye problems. The physician can selectively alter minute layers of eye tissue. Courtesy, Research to Prevent Blindness (see Chapter II). The lower view illustration shows a linear accelerator for the treatment of cancer. Courtesy, American Cancer Society (see Chapter II).

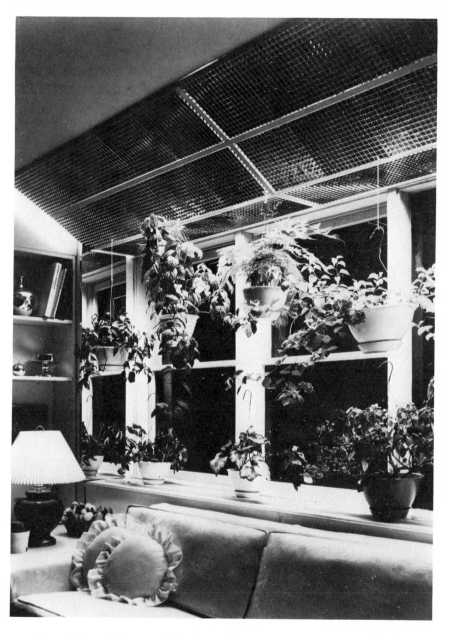

Plants thrive chiefly on visible light, with good reaction to red and blue wavelengths. Special fluorescent lamps are available for use indoors, making possible the pleasing hobby—or industry—of raising flowers without benefit of daylight. Duro-Lite photo (see Chapter II).

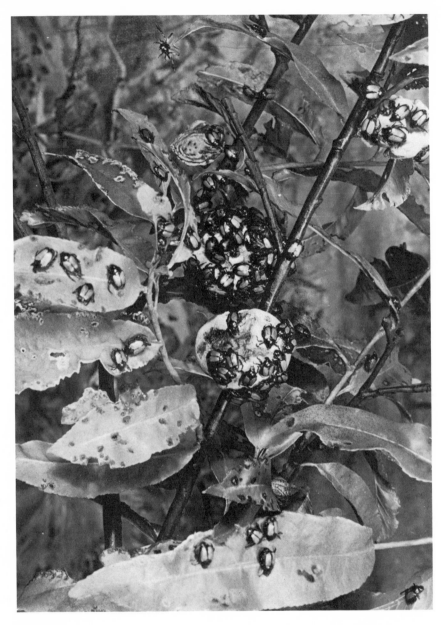

Insects such as beetles respond to different wavelengths than do human eyes. In general, red wavelengths are invisible, while blue and violet have greater attraction. Insect vision even extends into ultraviolet and shorter wavelengths, which cannot be seen by man. American Museum of Natural History photo (see Chapter II).

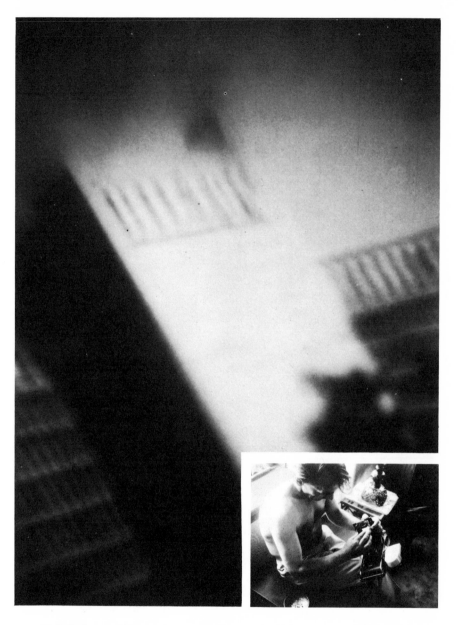

Ted Serios could stare into a camera and produce images such as those shown here. This involves the phenomenon of "thoughtography." (See Chapter III for a remarkable account by Dr. Jule Eisenbud, who submitted the photographs above.)

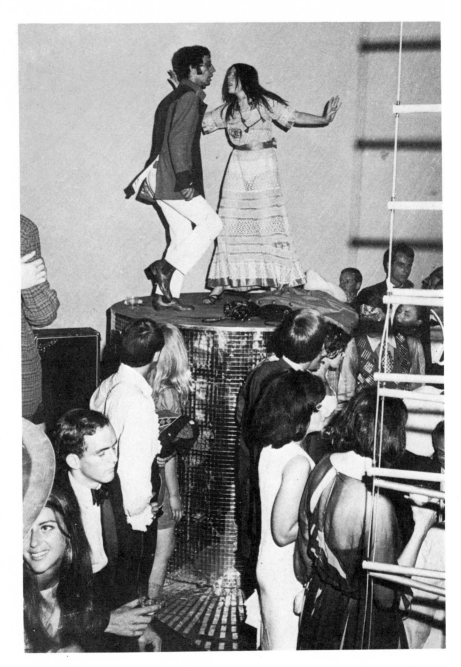

With the LSD cult of the late 60s and early 70s came the psychedelic age, in which brilliant color played a dominant role. A new world of color was discovered within the human psyche, and discotheques sprang up everywhere to feature color, sound, flashing lights. This view shows the Electric Circus, November 1970, in the East Village in New York. United Press International photo (see Chapter III).

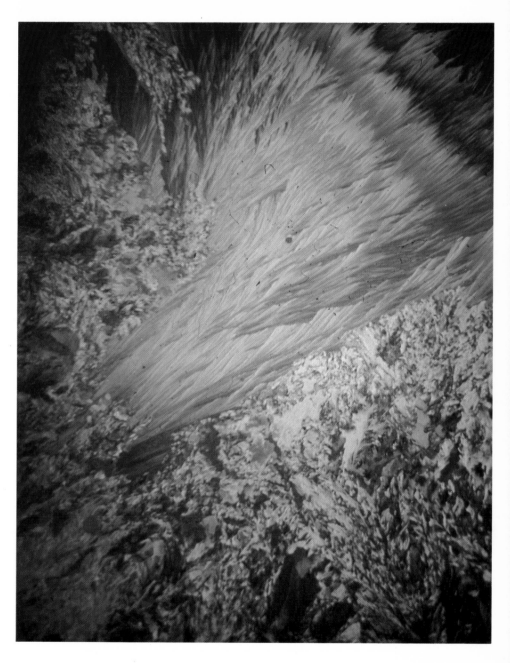

The type of abstract color effect used, in combination with music, by Cecil Stokes in Auroratone motion pictures to treat mentally depressed patients. By appealing to the two senses moods favorable to recovery were induced (see Chapter IV).

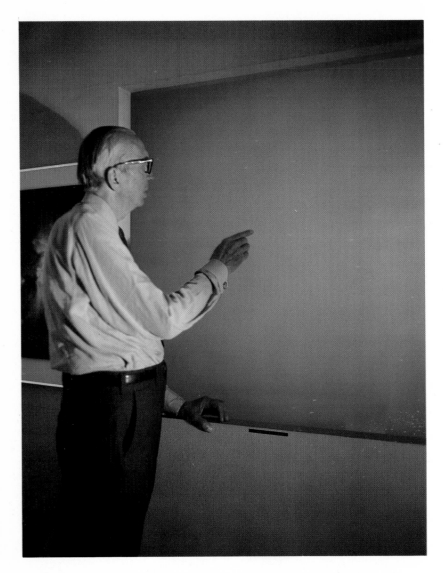

The stimulation of red and other warm colors tends to increase blood pressure, pulse, respiration. There is greater skin response (palmar conductance) and brain activity. Attention is directed outward toward the environment (see Chapter III).

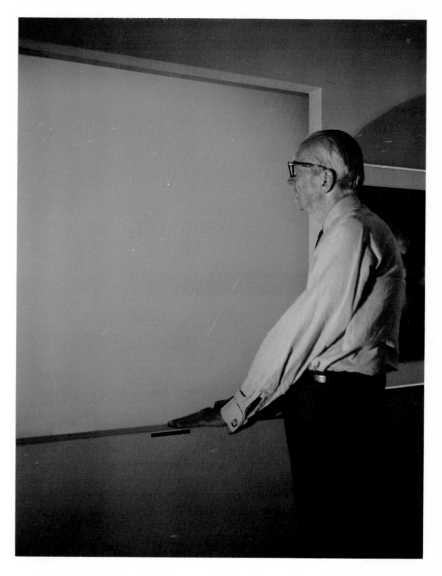

Green and blue tend to have a relaxing effect both physiologically and psychologically. The rate of body functions may be lowered, and there may be greater ability to concentrate inwardly, with less distraction from the environment (see Chapter III).

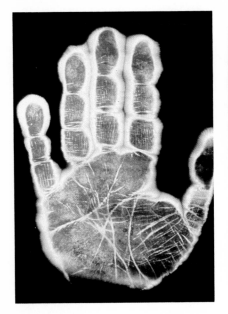

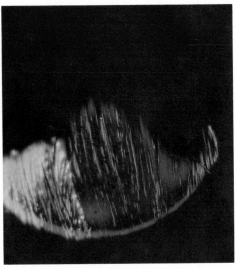

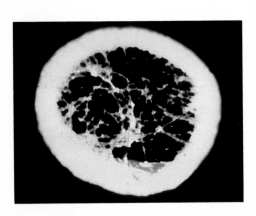

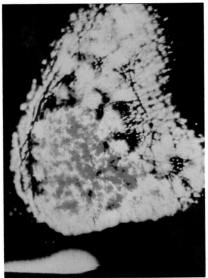

Examples of radiation-field photography (the Kirlian effect) from the laboratory of Thelma Moss of California. Shown above are high-voltage discharges of the hand and forehead. Below, from left to right, are coronas of a normal elbow and the elbow after accidental shock. Analyses of these bioenergetic fields show promise of revealing emotional moods and may serve as important revelations in medical diagnosis (see Chapter VI).

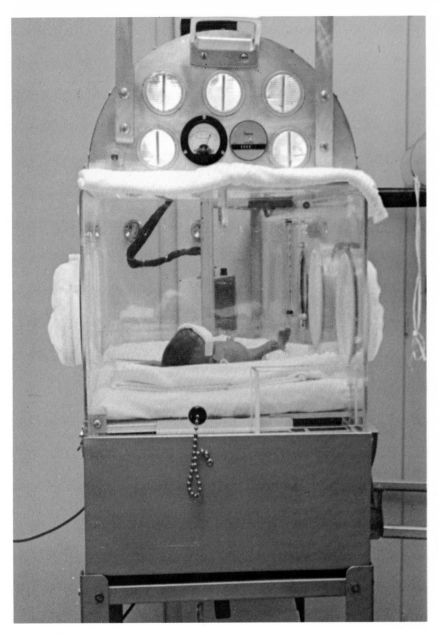

Phototherapy units employing blue light to treat pathologic jaundice (hyperbilirubinemia) in newborn infants. This is an effective example of visible-light therapy, uses for which are finding broader application (see Chapter VII).

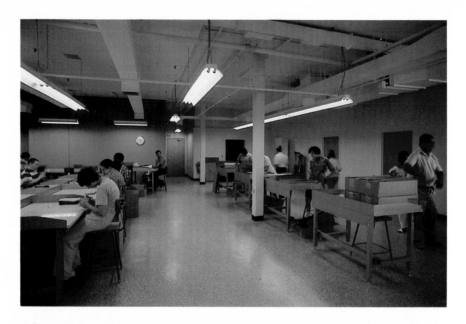

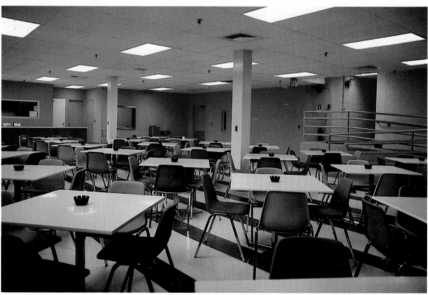

Color applications in a facility for the mentally retarded. By relieving glare and creating an emotionally pleasing environment work capacity is improved among handicapped persons who can do useful work and earn wages. Color variety also breaks up monotony and keeps spirits high (see Chapter VIII).

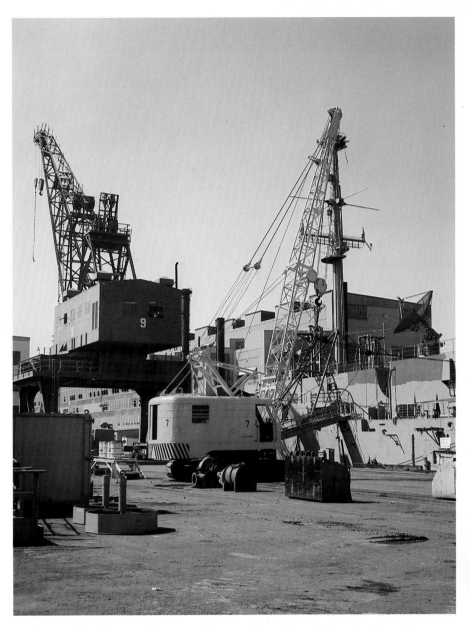

Use of safety colors in a navy shipyard. A specific code for color is mandatory practice for industry throughout America by the 1970 Occupational
Safety and Health Act (see Chapter VIII).

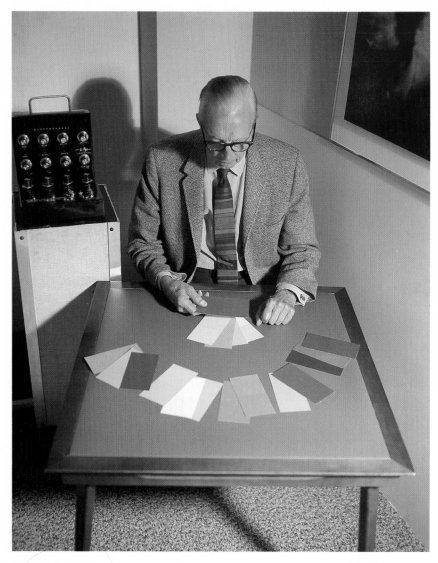

It is normal to prefer simple colors such as red and blue, followed by green and yellow. Preference shifts to neutral colors—brown, gray, black, white— may be indications of mental distress (see Chapter IX).

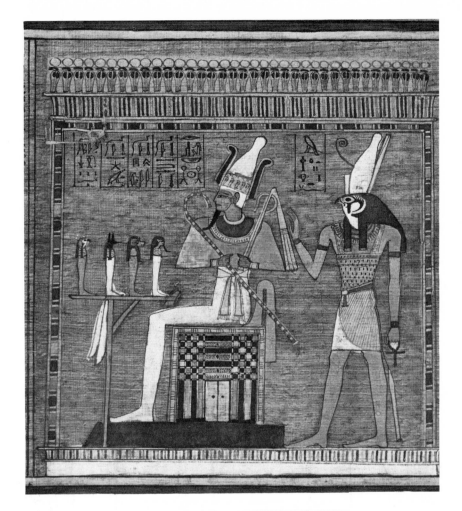

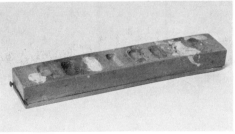

The top illustration from the Egyptian *Book of the Dead* shows Osiris (seated), his son Horus, and the four sons of Horus. Color is used symbolically. British Museum photo (see Chapter V). Below is an Egyptian paintbox used for decoration, c. 1450 B.C. Courtesy Metropolitan Museum of Art, Rogers Fund, 1948.

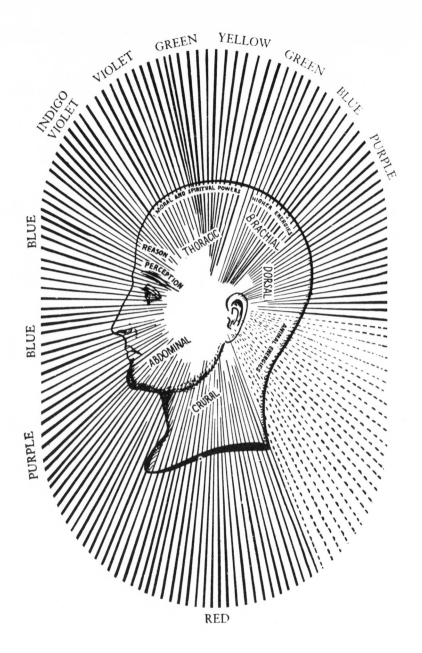

Odic (psychic) colors of the human brain as fancied by Minnie Weston and presented in Edwin D. Babbitt's celebrated book of 1878. Color emissions varied from person to person and revealed the quality of human minds (see Chapter VI).

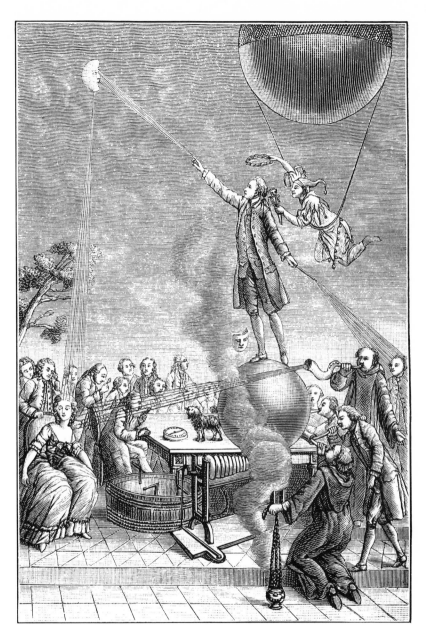

A 1784 engraving that satirizes the magnetic powers called upon by the great Franz Anton Mesmer to heal the ills of low-born as well as high-born Europeans. He commanded great fame and an uncertain reputation in his day (see Chapter VI).

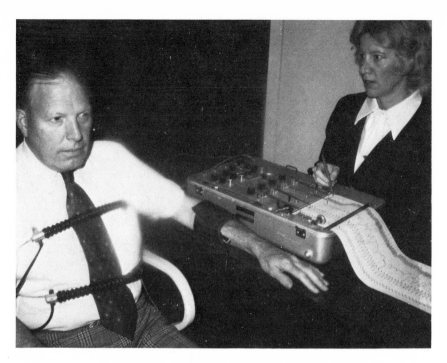

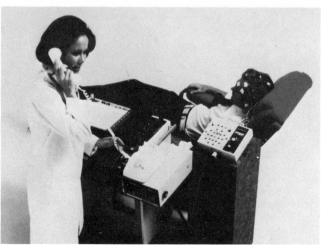

The top illustration shows the use of the polygraph to measure physiological reactions. Courtesy, American Polygraph Association (see Chapter VI). The lower view shows the use of the electroencephalograph (EEG) to measure brain waves. Courtesy, Beckman Instruments, Inc. (see Chapter VI).

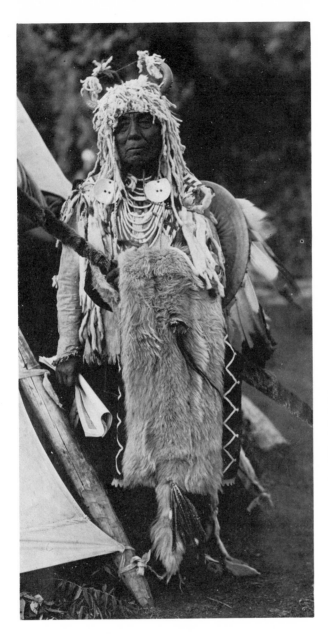

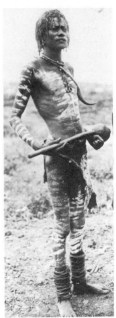

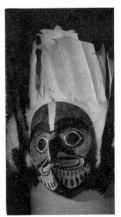

On the left a Umatilla medicine man with regalia. At top right a body-painted African native. At bottom right the headdress of a Tlingit Indian doctor of Alaska. There is color symbolism throughout. American Museum of Natural History photos (see Chapter VII).

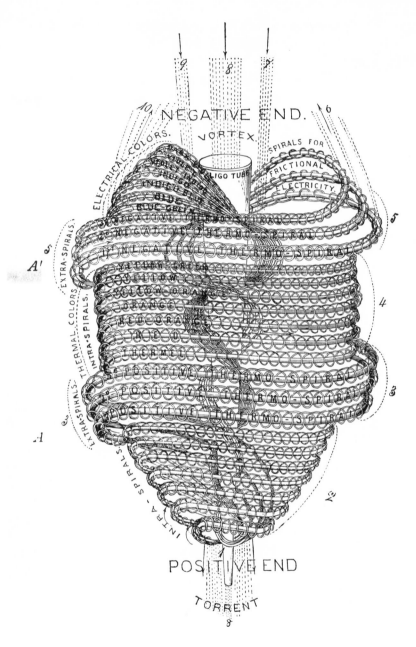

The general form of an atom as conceived by Edwin D. Babbitt in 1878. He remarkably foresaw the tremendous power associated with atomic energy and wrote effusively about it—as well as about color therapy (Chapter VII).

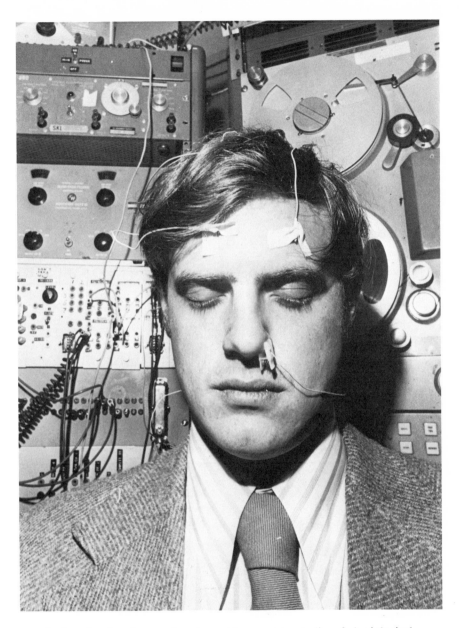

A view showing the use of equipment in computer studies of physiological changes that occur during transcendental meditation. Meditation promises many benefits but may also involve hazards. United Press International photo (see Chapter VIII).

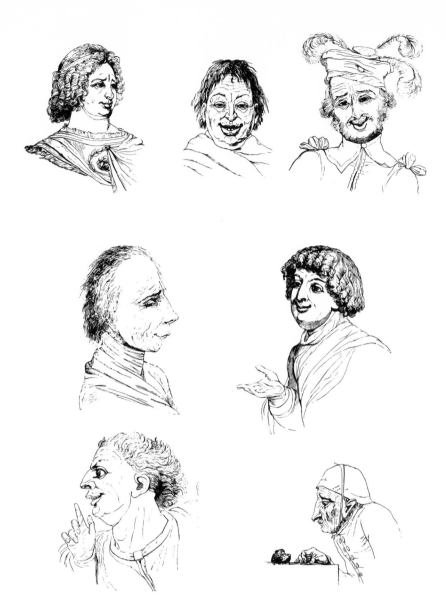

Colors readily lend themselves to personality types. Across the top from left to right might be green, red, purple. In the center from left to right might be yellow, blue. At bottom from left to right might be orange, brown. Portraits are 19th-century interpretations of *The Characters of Theophrastus,* a disciple of Aristotle who lived in the 4th century B.C.

overlap between the associations between color and feeling states and the associations between color and brain waves . . . suggests the possibility that subjective activity relating to colors may originate from the same underlying neuronal processes as do the brain waves. . . . I tend to favor the concept that the brain cell, neuronal, response to color came first, since in my studies and those of others the brain electrical response to red is one of alerting or arousal, whereas the brain electrical response to blue is one of relaxation. This happens in animals as well as man." As of this writing biofeedback techniques have lost some of their charm. Many practitioners, clinical groups, sectional and regional meetings have been dissolved. Yet biofeedback has become an affair of great interest to diagnostic and therapeutic medicine, and it no doubt will continue to be investigated in the future.

The aura, skin response, brain response—and also heartbeat, respiration, blood pressure—seem to be involved with color through electrical impulses. The ancient mystic or shaman, the faith healer, the modern psychiatrist and clinical psychologist, all have been and should be concerned with the rainbow that surrounds all beings. Fable is being supported by fact. The world is colorful inside and out.

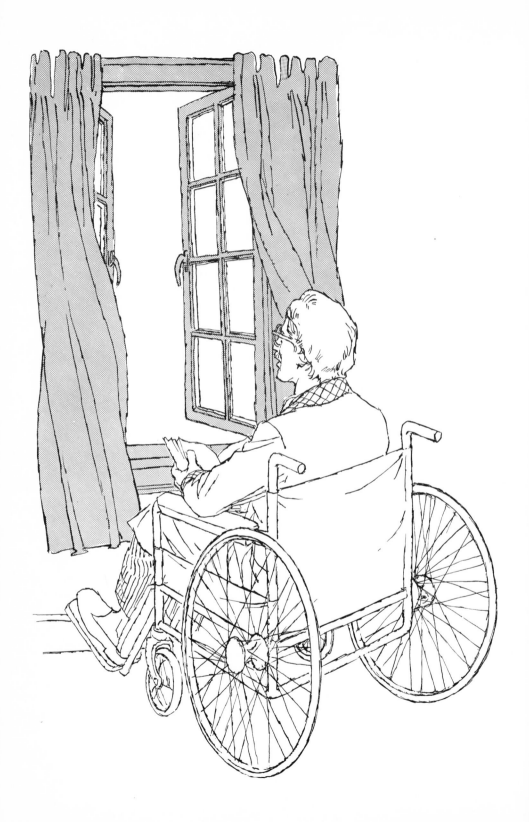

VII. To Heal The Body

Men have believed in the healing power of color since the beginning of recorded time and probably before. The reason is perhaps quite simple: sunlight sustains all life, and there is death without it. Even creatures that are able to survive in total darkness need foods that come from sunlit areas. The early chapters of this book review ancient traditions, symbolism, mythology, and superstitions related to color. This chapter gives special attention to the art of healing, both old and new.

ANCIENT TIMES

Color in healing has had its ups and downs over the centuries. The physicians of old revered it, believed in its healing properties, diagnosed through color, and prescribed color. In the age of enlightenment color healing survived but mostly through the loyalty of the mystic. Modern medical science later renounced color but not for long, as this chapter will relate, for its efficacy has lately restored it to grace. In the recognized science of photobiology, for example, there is promise of new therapies and new approaches to many of the maladies of life.

Worship of the sun and of light has forever intrigued man. The nature of diseases that shook the body, caused sores and fevers, spread in plagues, and brought death was unknown for the simple reason that the existence of microbes and viruses was unknown due to the lack of devices that could reveal them in magnification. All manner of therapies were applied, from chemicals to organic and inorganic potions to amulets and above all to pleas, sacrifices, and supplications to the gods.

In the Papyrus Ebers of the Egyptians, dating back to 1500 B.C., there are numerous references to colored minerals such as malachite and red and yellow clay. There is also reference to a poultice of raw meat for a black eye, to a red cake for constipation, to vermilion writing fluid mixed with goat's fat and honey to salve a wound. The Zoroastrians of ancient Persia practiced a form of color therapy based on the emanations of light.

PRIMITIVE VIEWS

Before proceeding to an orderly review of modern medical practice beginning with the great Hippocrates I shall mention witch doctors, medicine men, shamans, and the host of magic healers who still practice today—and actually outnumber the graduate medics of western civilizations!

Shamanism is identified with the primitive peoples of North and South America, with Eskimos, Lapps, and natives of the Far East and South Pacific. They function as priests, soothsayers, exorcists, doctors. They engage in bloodletting, kneading, hypnotism. They use herbs, nostrums, amulets and are familiar with curative drugs such as quinine and narcotics such as peyote. They wear gaudy costumes, dressing as bears, eagles, beavers, lions, and tigers. They carry beads, rattles, and wands and claim divine powers. Anthropologists have written of shamans, and works like *The Golden Bough* of Sir James George Frazer are replete with color lore.

Illness was the evil curse of demons and had to be driven out by the medicine man not only with incantations but with medicines taken from nature. He could contort his body, shake rattles, blow into the face of the ill one. The Navajos used white, red, yellow, blue, black paints in their curing practices. Some of the medicine men were skilled artists and made sand paintings of great beauty to call upon the favor of the gods. There were elaborate ceremonies associated with color that concerned birth, death, marriage, the slaying of men and animals, the summoning of sun or rain.

CHARMS AND AMULETS

It was assumed that, because disease came mysteriously out of nature, things from nature, color included, were necessary to combat it. What today may be looked upon as mere jewelry was once probably an amulet of protection as well as an item of adornment. The evil eye could be diverted and thwarted with bits of turquoise, blue beads, a daub of red or black on the forehead, red ribbon, a piece of coral. E. A. Wallis Budge in his *Amulets and Superstitions* writes: "In the bazaars of Cairo and Tanttah large blue-glazed pottery beads, fully half an inch in diameter, used to be sold to caravan men, who made bandlets of them and tied them to the foreheads of their camels before they set out on their journeys across the desert. The natives believed that the baleful glances of the evil eye would be attracted to the beads, and averted from the animals. . . . It is tolerably certain that the brass bosses and ornaments which decorate the harness of cart horses and shire-stallions were, like the great brass horns which rise from their collars, originally intended to protect the animal from the evil eye; but this fact has been forgotten, and amulets have degenerated into mere ornaments."

In other books of mine I have listed old superstitions that center around gems. Amber was for earache or eye troubles. Amber beads were for fever, rheumatism, toothache, headache. Amethyst was for gout. Carnelian restrained hemorrhage. Chalcedony was for gallstones. Emerald was for eye diseases, garnet for skin eruptions. Jade was for dropsy— and good at easing childbirth. Jet was for epilepsy. Ruby dipped in water was used as a stomachic. As late as 1948 a United Press International correspondent reported on the "pharmacy" of a hospital in Hyderabad, India, which included prescriptions involving gold, crushed pearls, emeralds, and rubies. A doctor at the hospital reported: "We make use of medical secrets that have been proved successful by the ages. Our theories are the siftings of Mogul, Persian, Greek, Roman, Egyptian, Hindu and Arab medical knowledge. We ourselves cannot always explain why our medicines work. But they have been working for centuries."

Prescribed also might be fungus from a grave, dew from grass, the organs of cold-blooded and warm-blooded creatures, plants shaped like a hand (for the hand) or like a tooth (for the tooth). Today there is still a sizable market for Chinese ginseng, said to prolong life and to serve as an aphrodisiac, among other marvels.

SUPERSTITIONS TODAY

There are people today who fear black cats, yellow in a theater; who wear blue as a bride, fill the English language with references to blackguards, red-letter days, blue gloom, green with envy, purple with rage, a brown taste in the mouth, yellow heathen. Not too long ago some physicians wore scarlet cloaks. Red flannel was used for scarlet fever and sore throat. To quote Budge: "A considerable number of rings made of red jasper, red faience, and red glass have been found in the tombs of Egypt; all are uninscribed and all have a gap in them. How and why they were used is not known, but a recent view about them is that they were worn as amulets by soldiers and by men whose work or duties brought them into conflict with their enemies, to prevent them from being wounded, or if wounded, to stop the flow of blood. It is possible that they were worn by women to prevent bleeding."

ORIGINS OF MODERN MEDICINE

Modern medicine usually credits Hippocrates (460?–370? B.C.) as its founder. He was less concerned with mysteries than with human habits and diets, the beating of men's hearts, and the pallor of the skin, thereby establishing a diagnostic and scientific attitude toward the ills of men. M.D. graduates today still take an oath attributed to him.

In the first century A.D. Aurelius Cornelius Celsus wrote eight books on medicine. His attitude toward color was practical and rational rather than occult. Medicines were prescribed with color in mind. A wide variety of flowers were prescribed—violet, iris, narcissus, rose, lily—and plasters in black, green, red, white. He wrote of red, "There is one plaster almost of a red color, which seems to bring wounds very rapidly to cicatrize." Of yellow, "Saffron ointment with iris-oil applied to the head, acts in procuring sleep, and in tranquilizing the mind."

Galen (130?–200? A.D.) was court physician to Marcus Aurelius among other famous Romans. He wrote some 500 treatises, lectured, taught, experimented, dissected. His authority in medicine was virtually undisputed for a number of centuries. Galen was attracted to color and declared, "I have been anointed with the white ointment of the tree of life." Color changes were significant in the diagnosis of disease. Here is one of his queries: "How, then, could blood ever turn into bone without having first become, as far as possible, thickened and white? And how could bread turn into blood without having gradually parted with its whiteness and gradually acquired redness?"

In the Dark Ages the seat of progress in medicine passed from Rome to Islam. Avicenna (980–1037?), an Arabian who spent most of his life in Persia, wrote the *Canon of Medicine*, a masterpiece of its time, and it gave him a great reputation until the Middle Ages. Color appeared everywhere in Avicenna's writings. There was diagnostic significance in the color of hair, flesh, eyes, urine, excrement. He developed a chart in which color was related to human temperament and to the physical condition of the body. Like earlier physicians, he was concerned with humors, or fluids of the body. He wrote: "Even imagination, emotional states and other agents cause the humors to move. Thus, if one were to gaze intently at something red, one would cause the sanguineous humor to move. This is why one must not let a person suffering from nose-bleeding see things of a brilliant red color." Blue soothed the movement of humors. Like Celsus before him, flowers were an intimate part of his remedies. Red flowers cured diseases of the blood, while yellow flowers cured diseases of the biliary system.

A RETURN TO THE MYSTIC

The logic of Hippocrates, Celsus, Galen, Avicenna—the study of objective and purely scientific evidence of disease—lost out during the Middle Ages. To the fore came a fraternity of mystics and alchemists who talked of harmony with divine forces, of God, philosophy, natural laws.

Pertinent to this brief story of color in the history of medicine is the name of Paracelsus (1493–1541), who publicly burned the works of Galen and Avicenna, declaring that disease was caused by disharmony with nature. Man was a composite of physical body, etheric body, astral body, ego, and a higher self. The Sun ruled his heart, the Moon his brain, Saturn his spleen, Mercury his lungs, Venus his kidneys, Jupiter his liver, and Mars his gall. The body of man was compounded of salt, sulphur, and mercury, and, if the balance of these elements was disturbed, illness followed. The genius and authority of Paracelsus became known throughout Europe. (He is still revered among mystics of today.) He cured with invocations, music, color, amulets, herbs, regulation of diet, bleeding, and purging.

Alchemy, the philosopher's stone, the elixir of life are a story in themselves. This prelude to modern chemistry boasts such names as Roger Bacon, Ben Johnson, Albertus Magnus, Thomas Aquinas, Nicholas Flamel, Raymond Lully, Jacob Böhme—and the aforementioned Paracelsus. Alchemy may have been devoted to the transmutation of metals, but beyond all it was a mystical and occult "science"—the philosopher's stone might be likened to Christ, a mixture of paganism and Christianity. Surviving today are magnificent manuscripts and tomes on alchemy, which intrigued Carl Jung as filled with profound and psychic revelations of what he termed the "collective unconscious," the mysteries of the universe, heaven and hell, and a possible regeneration of man himself.

Alchemy is replete with references to color. The principal hues were black, white, gold, and red. There were seven metals, related to seven planets, as well as eagles, salamanders, lions, crows, doves, swans, peacocks, flowers, all lending themselves to beauty and symbolism. The language of the alchemist was hidden in metaphors, its meanings made known only to initiates. Greatest of all achievements would be a true elixir of life, a red stone, potable gold, which could give everlasting life and freedom from disease. Today the dreams of the alchemist are becoming realities with the creation of plastics, precious stones, the amazing applications of electronic energy, the splitting of the atom.

THE FABULOUS DR. BABBITT

Out of the Renaissance and true to the sound principles of Hippocrates, Celsus, Galen, Avicenna came the science of medicine as it is known today: Vesalius, Harvey, Leeuwenhoek, Pasteur, Koch, Fleming; the microscope, the electronic microscope, x rays, radium, the laser, the diagnostic computer. Edwin D. Babbitt formed an interlude if not an interruption to the progress of enlightened medical and surgical practice. Babbitt stands as one of the most singular of men in the story of color therapy. He was both genius and charlatan, attacked, renounced, and disputed by the legal medical profession but adored by mystics.

Preceding Babbitt in the Victorian Age was General A. J. Pleasanton of Philadelphia, who in 1876 wrote a book, *Blue and Sun-Light,* in which he described a greenhouse with blue and clear panes of glass. He claimed to grow lush vines of grapes and experimented with pigs to increase their weight. To the General the blue sky held secrets to the bounty of life: it "deoxygenates carbonic acid gas, supplying carbon to vegetation and sustaining both vegetable and animal life with its oxygen."

A year later S. Pancoast wrote another book, *Blue and Red Light.* He attacked the medics of his time, praised the "Ancient Sages," and boasted of miraculous cures by passing rays of sunlight through red or blue glass. "In Life-unfoldment, the progress is from Black to Red—Red is the Zenith of manhood's prime; on the decline of Life the course is from Red to Black; in both unfoldment and decline, White is traversed, the healthful, elastic period of first maturity and of the medium stage of old age."

In the next year came the masterwork of Edwin D. Babbitt, *The Principles of Light and Color,* which created a worldwide if minor revolution in the art of color healing. (Let me make clear that I do not subscribe to Babbitt's theories. I have written about him, edited his book in 1967, and look upon him as one of the most colorful personalities in the broad and general field of color.) Babbitt was born in Hamden, New York on February 1, 1828, the son of a Congregational minister. (He died in 1905 and was the father of Irving Babbitt, writer on humanism and professor at Harvard.) He began adult life as a teacher, wrote and published books on penmanship, and took an interest in religion and "spiritual truths." At middle age, Babbitt declared himself a magnetist and psychophysician. He no doubt spent years in writing *The Principles of Light and Color*, which contained some 200,000 words and 560 pages. When it was published in 1878, Babbitt promptly became a famous man. Soon he headed a New York College of Magnetics. "Chromotherapy is based on eternal truth, and the sooner any great truth is adopted, the better it is for all concerned." This was a day of faith healers, patent medicines, magnetic belts, snake oil, and countless magic nostrums. Babbitt went into the business of color therapy and sold books, "Chromo Disks" and "Chromo Flasks," a "Thermolume" cabinet for color treatment, colored glass and filters, and a beautiful "Chromalume," designed as a 57-x-21-inch stained-glass window, to be placed within a house facing south and behind which persons could indulge in salubrious color treatments.

Babbitt built up a fantastic series of relationships between color and elements, color and minerals and spoke of such things as thermal colors and electrical colors. Let him speak in his own words. "There is a trianal series of graduations in the peculiar potencies of colors, the center and climax of electrical action, which cools the nerves, being in violet; the climax of electrical action, which is soothing to the vascular system, being in blue; the climax of luminosity being in yellow; and the climax of thermism or heat being in red. This is not an imaginary division of qualities, but a real one, the flame-red color having a principle of warmth in itself; the blue and violet, a principle of cold and electricity. Thus we have many styles of chromatic action, including progression of hues, of lights and shades, of fineness and coarseness, of electrical power, luminous power, thermal power, etc."

Concerning color therapy he wrote: "Red light, like red drugs, is the warming element of sunlight, with an especially rousing effect upon the blood and to some extent upon the nerves, especially as strained through some grades of red glass which will admit not only the red but the yellow rays, and thus prove valuable in paralysis and other dormant and chronic conditions." Yellow and orange stimulated the nerves. "Yellow is the central principle of nerve stimulus as well as the exciting principle of the brain which is the foundation head of the nerves." It was a laxative, an emetic, and a purgative. It was used by Babbitt in costiveness, bronchial difficulties, and hemorrhoids. Yellow mixed with considerable red was a diuretic. With a little red it was a cerebral stimulant. About half-and-half it was a tonic and helped the human system in general. Blue and violet had "cold, electrical and contracting potencies." The colors were soothing to all systems in which inflammatory and nervous conditions predominated—sciatica, hemorrhage of the lungs, cerebrospinal meningitis, neuralgic headache, nervousness, sunstroke, nervous irritability. Blue and white were particularly effective in sciatica, rheumatism, nervous prostration, baldness, and concussion. With rare prescience he described an atom, and in his book he made this remarkable statement: "If such an atom should be set in the midst of New York City, it must create such whirlwind that all its palatial structures, ships, bridges and surrounding cities, with nearly two millions of people, would be swept into fragments and carried into the sky."

To this day, a hundred years later, the chromotherapy of Babbitt still survives and is practiced. Books founded on his principles are still published. There are courses, lectures, meetings, schools of color, all traced to Babbitt. While his equipment, devices, and prescriptions cannot legally be manufactured or applied in the United States, chromotherapy is still a live "science" in England. If the reader is interested in this legerdemain, he should consult some of the books (mostly paperback) included in the bibliography: W. J. Colville, Corrine Heline, J. Dodson Hessey, Roland Hunt, C. E. Iredell (*Colour and Cancer*), S. G. J. Ouseley, C. G. Sander. *The Power of the Rays* by S. G. J. Ouseley, first printed in 1951, went into nine printings up to 1975. In it Babbitt is praised, and Ouseley does not hesitate to prescribe color treatments for ailments from asthma to epilepsy, diabetes, rheumatism, pneumonia, and mental disorders.

BORDERLINE PRACTICE

There will perhaps never be a sharp distinction between what is psychological in medicine and what is somatic and physical. As is said elsewhere in this book, there are psychic factors in disease as well as purely corporeal ones. The psychiatrist, who is concerned with human minds, spirits, and emotions, is just as necessary as the homeopathic physician and the surgeon, who are concerned with human bodies.

To mention a few borderline instances of color therapy for visible colors, red light has been used for erysipelas, scarlet fever, measles, eczema. Perhaps the red color of mercurochrome is effective in the healing of wounds partially because of its absorption of blue light. Red light has been said to reduce pain in postoperative incisions, acute inflammation, ultraviolet burn. Red (and infrared) produces heat in the tissues and dilates blood vessels. It may help to relieve the pains of rheumatism, arthritis, neuritis, lumbago. Blue has recent and vital applications, as will be described later. It has been prescribed for headaches, high blood pressure, and insomnia, perhaps because of its psychologically calming effects. Yellow, a cheerful color to the eye, has been said to stimulate appetite. Its rays have been found to raise low blood pressure associated with anemia, neurasthenia, and general debility—perhaps psychosomatically. Green has been neutral for the most part. As is said elsewhere, it is neutral in its effects on plants, and the same may be true of human beings.

MODERN MEDICAL PRACTICE

Let me shift from that which is mystical and probably questionable to the science of medicine as it is now recognized legally throughout America and the world, to doctors and practitioners with medical-school degrees and government-approved licenses.

Largely because of Babbitt and a vast clique of specious and fraudulent color healers the modern medical profession has disdained color as a therapeutic agent. There has been less indifference than outright hostility. The American Medical Association and the U.S. Post Office have denounced chromotherapists and put some of them out of business. Today, however, light and color are working their way back into the medical field. In a science known as photobiology the strange effects of light, visible and invisible, are being studied as they tend to influence or affect chemicals, living things, microbes, plants, animals, men. I have tried my best to keep abreast of research here and am happy to recount some of my findings herewith.

Modern medicine has acknowledged the value of infrared radiation, for example, which is useful in relieving certain aches and pains. The merits of ultraviolet are also acknowledged and have had therapeutic use, as is described later. In other realms of the complete electromagnetic spectrum therapeutic uses are found for short x rays, radium rays, and long rays, which are applied in diathermy. But what about *visible* light— red, yellow, green, blue? I quote from a few acceptable sources. "Knowledge of the significance of visible light as a healing agent is inversely proportional to the universal importance of visible light in biology."—Friedrich Ellinger. "Visible light, as much as UV or infrared radiation, has the ability to exert measurable biological effects. Medical uses of the visible spectrum have been virtually ignored by physicians for the past 90 years."—Thomas R. C. Sisson. "Visible light is apparently able to penetrate all mammalian tissues to a considerable depth; it has even been detected within the brain of a living sheep."—Richard J. Wurtman.

HELIOTHERAPY

Light and color as therapeutic agents had an early beginning, as Friedrich Ellinger describes: "Knowledge of the therapeutic action of light is one of mankind's oldest intellectual possessions. The earliest experiences depended of course upon nature's own light source, the sun. Sunbathing was practiced even long ago by the Assyrians, Babylonians and Egyptians. A highly developed sun- and air-bathing cult existed in ancient Greece and Rome. The old Germans regarded the healing powers of sunlight very highly and worshipped the rising sun as a deity. The Incas of South America also practiced a sun cult."

With the scientific progress of medicine the use of new diagnostic measures and devices, new chemicals, medicines, antibiotics, the old art of heliotherapy was neglected. In the nineteenth century a modern pioneer came upon the scene—and phototherapy was off to a new start. Niels R. Finsen of Denmark found magic in light. In his earlier years he sought to treat smallpox with visible red light to prevent scar tissue. Around 1896 he noted the actinic properties of sunlight and founded a Light Institute to deal with tuberculosis. For this he was honored with a Nobel prize in 1903. Sunlight became a chief therapy for tuberculosis, and sanitariums throughout the world were given architectural features of sun decks, sun parlors, and sun roofs.

Ultraviolet radiation is essential to human welfare. It helps to prevent rickets, stimulates vitamin-D formation, destroys germs, and creates a number of changes within the body. Yet too much of it can lead to skin cancer. According to W. F. Loomis, a biochemist, rickets is "the earliest air pollution disease." During the industrial revolution black smoke darkened the sky and rickets became an affliction of epidemic proportions in the cities of England and Europe. Once attributed to poor diet, it has been proved to be due to a deficiency of solar ultraviolet radiation. Infants born in the autumn were more likely to become rachitic than those born in spring.

A measure of ultraviolet light is undoubtedly needed in artificial environments, and sources emitting it are now being made. For years the Russians have been using ultraviolet radiation to supplement conventional fluorescent light in schools, hospitals, and offices. In schools children grow faster than usual, work ability and grades are improved, and catarrhal infections are fewer. Russian miners are required to take ultraviolet treatments. What takes place? According to a report of the International Commission on Illumination, "The action of ultraviolet radiation intensifies enzymatic processes of metabolism, increases the activity of the endocrine system, promotes the immunobiological responsiveness of the body and improves the tone of the central nerve and muscular system." This is a great deal. It may be noted parenthetically that, while it is favorable to the health of living things, ultraviolet can damage works of art, pigments, dyestuffs, and textiles. It thus may be good for schools but not for museums and art galleries. Incandescent light, which emits virtually no ultraviolet, is better. Further notes on ultraviolet and balanced light are given in Chapter II.

PHOTOSENSITIVITY

If ultraviolet light can tan the skin and cause erythema, visible light can also have effects. It is a strange fact, for example, that exposure to *visible* light can help to repair the damage of invisible *ultraviolet* light.

In a rare affliction known as *urticaria solare* some unfortunate souls will develop a skin rash if exposed to *visible* blue or violet light. The reason? Harold F. Blum explains that "It is safe to say that this response occurs in skins which are otherwise apparently normal, because of the presence of a photoactive substance which absorbs in the blue and violet regions of the spectrum."

Skin eruptions, occurring upon exposure to sunlight, may follow the use of cosmetics, perfumes, aftershave lotions. They may also follow ingestion of strawberries or buckwheat cakes. Workers have been known to have their skin break out after exposure to some industrial fumes, the handling of parsnips or figs, coal-tar products. Some animals may be fatally "burnt" by sunlight after eating certain plants, such as St. John's wort. Arthur C. Giese writes: "In some parts of Italy ... only black sheep can be kept, and in some parts of Arabia, only black horses. White patches on black horses are covered with black pigment."

While most of the above effects are unwanted and inimical, in phototherapy today the deliberate creation of light sensitivity is finding therapeutic applications. Some persons sensitive to ultraviolet or visible blue-violet in sunlight can be given a drug which effectively quenches the unwanted radiation and enable them to enjoy outdoor life on a sunny day. Psoriasis can be treated with dyes applied topically. In an infection known as *Herpes simplex* virus (cold sores) it has become comon practice to paint the affected area with dye and then to expose it to visible light. Various dye colors have been tried (the dyes themselves may be inert). One dye, chrome yellow in color, has been found particularly effective. To quote from an article by Joseph L. Melnick: "The therapy now in use consists of rupturing early vesicular lesions with a sterile needle, application of the proflavine dye solution to the base of the ruptured vesicles, and exposure for 30 minutes to a light source of proper wavelength (450nm for proflavine) and sufficient intensity. Re-exposure to the light is recommended 4 times during the next 2 days. If new lesions develop, the procedure is repeated." The color of the 450nm light source is a blue-violet. The proflavine dye is yellow.

In a recent article for *Photochemistry and Photobiology* (April 1977) a series of articles was devoted to the use of dyes for *Herpes simplex* virus. This affliction is quite prevalent, particularly in genital infections that follow venereal disease such as gonorrhea. Michael Jarrett reviews the subject, casts "doubt on the efficacy of neutral red and proflavine therapy," and favors proflavine *sulfate*, which has a yellowish color and absorbs highly in the blue-violet region of the visible spectrum. As a light source he chose incandescent light passing through a narrow-band filter (blue) over fluorescent light. He comments: "Photodynamic inactivation of *Herpes simplex in vitro* is enhanced at higher temperatures. Therefore the heat emitted by an incandescent source at close range makes the incandescent source theoretically a better choice in the clinical setting than a cool white fluorescent bulb."

The use of porphyrins has had favorable effects in the treatment of some superficial forms of cancer and tumors. Ivan Diamond and his associates in a talk for the American Society for Photobiology (June 1973) noted that "Malignant tumors take up and retain hematoporphyrin to a greater extent than normal tissue." With a tumor, for example, the sensitizing agent (the porphyrin) accumulates at the afflicted part and the cancerous area is "severely damaged when exposed to visible or near ultraviolet light." For the future "Photodynamic therapy offers a new approach to the treatment of brain tumors and other neoplasms resistant to existing forms of therapy." In another use of dye-sensitizing agents hematoporphyrin fluoresces to a red color when exposed to blue light. Where there may be malignant growth, states Thomas P. Vogl in an article in *Optics News*, "The suspected region, for example, the oral cavity, is exposed to blue light." The area will fluoresce and may "enable the surgeon to know what portions of tissue must be excised." It should be admitted that the relation of dyes, light, and skin afflictions is still under study and still subject to skepticism. More is being learned as time goes on.

VISIBLE BLUE LIGHT

One of the recent wonders of color in medicine is the use of visible blue light in the treatment of pathologic jaundice in newborn infants. Hyperbilirubinemia, pathologic jaundice, is unfortunately common among newborn infants. It may run as high as 17 percent in the *premature* baby. Red blood cells are decomposed, with bilirubin a result. A yellow substance accumulates, giving the baby a yellow-orange color. This can lead to deafness, brain damage, and impaired mental and muscular reactions. It may further cause cerebral palsy and even death.

Treatments such as blood transfusion formerly were applied but with little success. Around 1958 Dr. Richard J. Cremer of England noted, with his associates and nursing staff, that infants in bassinets near a window showed less jaundice than those located away from natural light. Infants with the affliction were then exposed moderately to sunlight, while experiments with artificial light were conducted. Through laboratory and clinical tests the most efficacious of all lights was a blue. From this a new therapy was developed. Special blue lamps having a narrow spectral emission (and completely free of ultraviolet) proved best. Today the method is widely used in America, Europe, and elsewhere.

Further studies are being conducted. How intense should the blue light be? How long should it be used and for how many periods? Could the light application be intermittent? Is blue superior to other colors? This last question has been dealt with by Dr. Thomas R. C. Sisson: "The presence of other wavelengths in the visible spectrum . . . does not increase the effectiveness of phototherapy." Dr. Sisson has two further points to make. First, the infant's eyes should be protected against excessive radiation. Second, where the special blue lamps were used in a hospital nursery for premature infants, nurses "complained of discomfort or even nausea." To relieve this, a few gold lamps were introduced.

Perhaps these are new beginnings. The magical properties of light and color, granted by men since the earliest of times, accepted, renounced, and accepted again through the ages, have forever held fascination. The fact that they have such strong emotional appeal has been to their advantage. But this at the same time has raised skepticism. Both the emotional and the physical aspects of color are now being acknowledged as having therapeutic potential. It would be delightful, of course, if a thing of such psychological beauty—color—also held a mundane role in human physiological wellbeing.

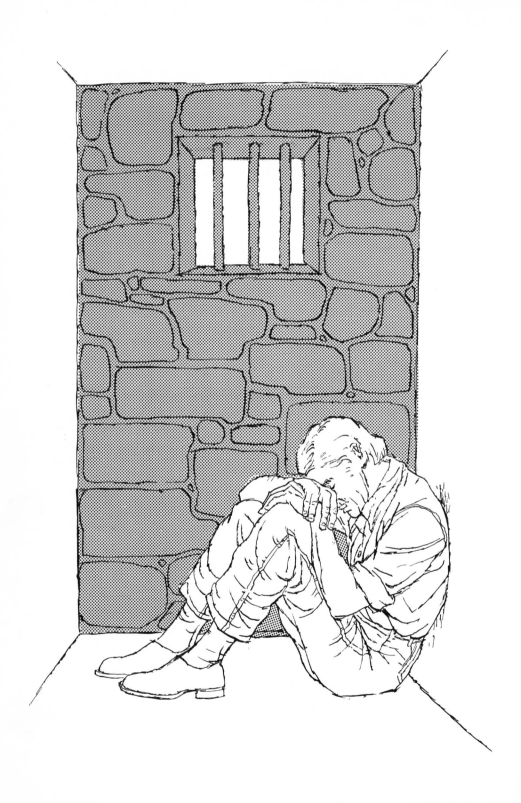

VIII. To Calm The Mind

M. D. Vernon has made a statement that in my opinion may be accepted as a basic law in the application of color to human environments: *"Thus we must conclude that normal consciousness, perception and thought, can be maintained only in a constantly changing environment."* Vernon goes on to remark, "Where there is no change, a state of 'sensory deprivation' occurs; the capacity of adults to concentrate deteriorates, attention fluctuates and lapses, and normal perception fades. In infants who have not developed a full understanding of their environment, the whole personality may be affected, and readjustment to a normal environment, may be difficult."

SENSORY DEPRIVATION IN ANIMALS

Vernon's conclusion, which relates to consciousness, perception, and thought, also applies to physical wellbeing, for if there is severe visual monotony, the body may in turn be adversely troubled. Man is living more and more in environments of his own design and control. While this sad state of affairs is becoming increasingly common for human beings, many animals have been so isolated for ages.

While caged animals, protected from predators and natural enemies, can live a life of secure ease, bliss is rarely encountered. Confinement and monotony may lead the animal to starve itself, to overeat, to refuse to procreate, and to devour and destroy its kind or any other kind. Apes have been observed to withdraw within themselves in the manner of schizophrenics if left alone or surrounded by blank walls. Other creatures may lapse into a fatal lethargy. Zoos are rapidly building better and more spacious environments with splendid results. Cubs are being born to parents who previously refused to breed in more austere captivity. Life spans are increasing. No doubt important lessons are being learned for days in the future when man too will be an enclosed mortal who will need not only proper food, light, and exercise but also agreeable visual sights and colors to help him maintain a sane normality.

On the effect of light and illumination John Ott tells of an experience at the Burnett Park Zoo in Syracuse, New York. To protect against vandalism, floodlights were installed. The result? Spring had arrived! "The zoo has been turned into a veritable maternity ward. The cougars fell in love all over again and produced their fourth litter. We collected five goose eggs. At least eight lambs were born, and the deer population increased by twenty. Big Lizzie gave birth to a bear cub. The wallaby produced a new mini-kangaroo and the chimpanzee is expecting in August."

Balanced, full-spectrum lighting has also had remarkable effects. Jozef Laszlo of the Houston Zoological Gardens in Texas has reported on the effect of full-spectrum fluorescent light on reptiles and amphibians. Some snakes and lizards had short life spans, and he suspected that lack of exposure to sunlight was inimical. Laszlo installed fluorescent tubes with good emission throughout the spectrum, including a small amount of ultraviolet. (The tubes were Vita-Lite, made by the Duro-Test Corporation of New Jersey.) Laszlo soon noted that the animals became more active. Some of the snakes, long starved, took food. One specimen that had refused to eat had its appetite restored after less than two weeks. He commented, "As a result of these trials and experiments, we concluded that the radiation and intensity from an undistorted visible spectrum lamp may be more important for the maintenance of this specimen, and others, than middle and long wave ultraviolet alone, or of ultraviolet in combination with a distorted visible spectrum lamp."

SENSORY DEPRIVATION IN HUMAN BEINGS

Sensory deprivation is an intriguing subject. Because of man's increasing existence within artificial environments physiologists, psychiatrists, psychologists are devoting attention to the effects of isolation. Books are written and conferences held. Isolation has been suffered in the past by caged animals, prisoners in solitary confinement, "shunning" in some religious sects, hazing, in which persons are punished by being ignored, the habits of hermits and monks. In modern society isolation may characterize people confined in hospitals for broken bones or heart attacks, the insane, the old, astronauts and aquanauts, aviators, men working at automated machines. R. L. Gregory writes, "It seems that in the absence of sensory stimulation, the brain can run wild and produce fantasies which may dominate."

Brainwashing has in part relied on forced isolation, which tends to break the spirit. Curiously, the effects of isolation may at times resemble the effects that follow ingestion of hallucinogenic drugs. Three Canadian scientists, Woodburn Heron, B. K. Doane, and T. H. Scott, report: "It is unlikely that the effects observed after isolation can be attributed merely to the forgetting of perceptual habits during the isolation period. They seem to resemble somewhat the effects reported after administration of certain drugs (such as mescaline and lysergic acid) and after certain types of brain damage. When we consider as well the disturbances which occurred during isolation (for example, vivid hallucinatory activity), it appears that exposing the subject to a monotonous sensory environment can cause disorganization of brain function similar to, and in some respects as great as, that produced by drugs or lesions." Among the disturbed brain functions are impairment of color perception, hallucinations involving color, and the distortion of color images.

EARLY CANADIAN FINDINGS

Concentrated studies of sensory deprivation were made in Canada during the 50s. In *The Psychology of Perception* M. D. Vernon describes a number of clinical studies on the effects of a monotonous environment. Here is one example: "Under the direction of Hebb, at the University of McGill, experiments were carried out to investigate the effects of keeping people for periods up to five days in a completely homogenous and unvarying environment. In a small room they lay on a bed; they heard nothing but the monotonous buzz of machinery; they had translucent goggles over their eyes so that they could see only a blur of light; and they wore long cuffs which came down over their hands and prevented their touching anything. Some observers were able to stay in these surroundings continuously for five days; others could not endure them for more than two days."

Professor Vernon comments that at first the subjects slept a great deal, but after about a day they could sleep only in snatches. They became bored and restless, unable to concentrate. "In fact, when their intelligence was tested, it was found to have deteriorated. They frequently suffered from visual and auditory hallucinations. When they emerged from their incarceration, their perceptions of their surroundings were impaired. Objects appeared blurred and unstable; straight edges, such as those of walls and floors, looked curved; distances were not clear; and sometimes the surroundings moved and swirled round them, causing dizziness." This surely suggests the need for reasonable exposure to color and other sensations in an environment. It also points out the need for variety. Blank surfaces tend to fade out if viewed continuously. Even colors may fade into neutral gray. Vision seems to degenerate unless stimulated, and the mind itself drops into lethargy.

INFANTS AND HOSPITAL PATIENTS

Professor Vernon describes a study conducted by H. R. Schaffer on infants under seven months of age who were hospitalized for periods of one to two weeks. Schaffer reports that the environment of the hospital was monotonous, lacking variation. On being taken home the infants continued to stare into space with blank expressions on their faces. Such behavior persisted for a few hours or a couple of days.

Herbert Leiderman and fellow researchers have written of further hazards of isolation that center around medical care. Hospitals in particular need color as well as other sensory interests such as music, television, and visitors. Leiderman and his group studied volunteers who willingly confined themselves up to 36 hours in a respirator in which they were able to see only a small area of ceiling. Only five of seventeen could endure the confinement for the full 36 hours. "All reported difficulty in concentration, periodic anxiety feelings and a loss of ability to judge time. Eight . . . reported some distortions of reality, ranging from pseudo-somatic delusions to frank visual hallucinations. Four subjects terminated the experiment because of anxiety; two of these in panic tried to release themselves forcibly from the respirator."

What is highly pertinent here is that disturbed or ill people, not to mention sane ones and cooped-up apartment dwellers, are often expected to spend long hours and days in confined and drab quarters. Assuming that a surgical operation may correct a man's illness, what if his confinement then leads to other and unexpected maladies? Leiderman and his group write: "If normal persons can develop psychoticlike states . . . how much more likely it is that sick patients, perhaps already perilously near the mental breaking point, can be tipped into psychopathological states by the stress of sensory deprivation. Delirium may be imminent for patients weakened by fever, toxicity, metabolic disturbance, organic brain disease, drug action or severe emotional strain; sensory deprivation may tip the balance. We have accumulated clinical evidence that sensory deprivation may be one element of importance in the etiology of mental disturbance as a complication of various medical and surgical conditions."

SPACE TRAVEL

A symposium held in 1957 by the American Psychological Association had the title "Sensory deprivation: facts in search of a theory." In most scientific work the emphasis is usually the opposite: a search of facts. Innumerable "facts" about isolation can be quoted, but how can one make sense out of them? Marvin Zuckerman writes, "The sensory deprivation (SD) experiment is a nightmare to the experimentalist who craves clearcut, well-controlled experimental situations."

I have a reason for devoting considerable time to sensory deprivation, for in my profession as a color consultant I am frequently called upon to write lighting and color specifications for facilities housing or accommodating groups of people. What is the best way to assure their welfare and efficiency? Any observations or "facts" that I can assemble are thus of definite interest and value to me.

Perhaps space travelers, busy as they are with instruments, radio instructions, and the like, will be kept sufficiently occupied so as not to be affected by the monotony of their crowded capsule. Yet passengers with little or nothing to do might well encounter no end of mental distress. Just about everyone has been cornered somewhere at one time, in a stalled train, a doctor's office, an airport or a hotel on a rainy day. Patience will collapse in a few hours. But how about days if not weeks?

The National Aeronautics and Space Administration in its Tektite program has undertaken a series of experiments in "habitability assessment." Two giant cylinders placed fifty feet under water in the Virgin Islands in the Atlantic Ocean have been occupied and inhabited by various groups of aquanauts for periods of fourteen, twenty, and thirty days. All were well qualified for the ordeal, tested psychologically and rated above average as engineers and intelligent human beings. All had duties to perform that left little time for loneliness or boredom. The two things that they missed most were lack of news and lack of privacy. Much of their leisure time was spent in conversation and in listening to taped music.

Some quotations from a report prepared by David Nowlis, Harry H. Watters, and Edward C. Wortz, who undertook a special assignment on habitability for NASA, are pertinent. "Aquanauts explicitly and spontaneously stated in a number of interviews that they themselves were surprised at how little anxiety they felt during the mission. . . . Most complaints centered around the general area of habitat design. Specifically, the aquanauts were dissatisfied with the design of the habitat affecting the performance of their tasks. . . . Although crewmen reported books as their favorite pastime, they did not spend much of their time reading them." Perhaps this was a matter of giving answers that are expected! The participants missed spouses and families. They liked music and TV films. They least liked cooking and did not seem to miss fresh air. The report continues: "With respect to moods, it is clear that the positive moods of social affection, pleasantness, activation and concentration tend to decline dramatically with increase in mission duration. This suggests that, along with the dramatic decline in positive feeling, there is a tendency for these moods to be replaced by a state of flat and steady unemotionality. Apparently, longer missions encourage aquanauts to be in a routinized, neutral mood where there is less activation, less concentration and less intensity of feeling either in a positive or negative sense."

The National Aeronautics and Space Administration has more recently conducted similar experiments with women to determine their ability to withstand long periods of inaction and isolation. Paid volunteers of medium age (35 to 45) were expected to adjust to a horizontal and virtually immobile position for some 24 days! The confined space was windowless and soundproof. Although they lay in a supine position, they exercised on a bicycle contraption, rested on their elbows when eating, and slipped into a horizontal shower and toilet compartment. They could read lying down by wearing prism lenses. Their reactions were monitored, with particular attention to anxiety. Cycles of sixteen hours of light and eight hours of darkness were arranged. The women confessed to great boredom, weakness, vertigo, and to some psychological distress, but they survived the test well and could undoubtedly become space travelers in the future. Isolation, however, can have far more serious consequences than such experiments suggest. Not all people are young, eager to venture into space, or specially trained for technical and scientific missions.

PEACE AND QUIET

Many people harbor the delusion that they could perform great creative work if only they could find a place of "peace and quiet!" Henry David Thoreau might be an exception, but genius is usually accompanied by an exhausting and frenzied capacity for hard work. Men such as Dickens, Dostoevski, Mozart, Van Gogh and numerous others performed remarkable work for several reasons: to earn money, to meet deadlines, or to stifle an inner and fervid drive. To sit in a cottage by the sea or amid forests, mountains, flower gardens may make nature unbearable to even the most dedicated soul. In some experiments on sensory deprivation persons have planned to occupy their minds with constructive reflections. Alas, those who may plan to do some creative thinking may soon find that they have no desire to concentrate. Instead their thoughts drift through their minds in random sequence. Which leads to the currently popular subject of meditation.

Meditation, biofeedback, mind control are popular subjects today. There are biofeedback research societies, clinics, private practitioners, books, courses, instruments, blending oriental philosophies and modern scientific investigations. Barbara Brown writes: "The anxieties of human beings are imbedded in the not-knowing of their own insides. . . . By this writing hundreds of studies have confirmed the fact that when human beings can perceive their own brain wave alpha activity they can learn to control it."

Color is involved here. As has been noted, if monotony is forced upon a person, voluntarily or involuntarily, sensory deprivation may result. People might be better able to cope with this if they could learn to meditate, to control their functions, physical as well as mental and psychological. There are reservations, however, for, as has been said, *it is a normal and natural condition for all the senses to be stimulated continually if moderately: a condition of absolute peace is unnatural even in sleep!* The paradox is that isolation can have ill effects, yet, if it is deliberately accepted and controlled, it can have many therapeutic benefits.

Meditation may not be for everyone. Yet mind-training courses have been taken by thousands of hopeful mortals, often with excellent results. If a person, through anxiety or other distress, finds comfort and relief in meditation, this is all to the good. Yet this writer confesses to a certain skepticism and prejudice. Some people who take mind-training courses become neurotic. There may be danger in burrowing too deeply into one's psyche. There may be quite the opposite of the "kingdom of heaven" within. Gary E. Schwartz writes in *Psychiatry and Mysticism* that "The nervous system needs reasonably intense and varied external stimulation, and there is no evolutionary, ethological, or biological precedent for massive and prolonged meditation."

Mind training, mind control, biofeedback sometimes rely on hypnosis, which may cause problems. Some people who have posed as mystics or spiritual leaders have used hypnosis as a technique. If phenomenal results have been achieved at times, so also has backlash caused reverse and adverse effects. I do not want to disparage meditation entirely, however, as it can have beneficial effects. Through the control of alpha and theta waves by voluntary concentration (and as recorded by professional biofeedback instruments) various favorable therapeutic results may follow. By lessening anxiety and tension high blood pressure (hypertension) may be relieved if not cured. There may be benefits for those troubled by depression, insomnia, or addiction to alcohol and drugs.

TOGETHERNESS

If there is danger in being alone, too much "togetherness" may also cause trouble. In small groups of people some persons seek privacy and withdrawal. Confinement in spaceships, submarines, institutions, dormitories often pits friend against friend. Admiral Byrd, in his book *Alone*, writes: "Even at Little America I knew of bunkmates who quit speaking because each suspected the other of inching his gear into the other's allotted space; and I knew of one who could not eat unless he could find a place in the mess hall out of sight of the Fletcherist who solemnly chewed his food twenty-eight times before swallowing. In a polar camp little things like that have the power to drive even disciplined men to the edge of insanity. During my first winter at Little America I walked for hours with a man who was on the verge of murder or suicide over imaginary persecutions by another man who had been his devoted friend. For there is no escape anywhere. You are hemmed in on every side by your own inadequacies and the crowding pressures of your associates. The ones who survive with a measure of happiness are those who can live profoundly off their intellectual resources." Note the last sentence. If a person would seek peace and happiness in meditation—which might well lead to sensory deprivation—he might be better advised to develop his "intellectual resources."

THE PRACTICAL SPECIFICATION OF COLOR

How to apply color to such facilities as offices, industrial plants, schools, hospitals, mental institutions, convalescent and retirement homes? Let me end this chapter with suggestions and recommendations from my own experience.

LIGHTING

Artificial light should preferably be neutral and slightly warm in quality. If a modest amount of longwave UV can be added, so much the better. For the best appearance of human complexion, furnishings, food, the light source should be well balanced in its emission of red, yellow, green, blue, violet. If there are gaps, some objects in the environment may have an ungainly look. High levels of illumination may be unnecessary except where difficult eye tasks are to be performed.

BRIGHTNESS

Except for ceilings white or off-white *should not be used on walls* where groups of persons are assembled. High environmental brightness not only handicaps seeing (by introducing a form of interior "snow" blindness) but also severely constricts the pupil opening of the human eye, an action that is muscular and very fatiguing. Prolonged exposure to high brightness can also cause damage to the visual organ. As has been said in Chapter III, it can aggravate muscular imbalance, refractive difficulties, nearsightedness, and astigmatism, not to overlook eye congestions and inflammation. Avoid conflicting areas of severe brightness differences, which may force the eye to undergo tiring muscular adjustments.

COLOR REACTIONS

There is wide latitude here. If the color (and brightness) covers the general field of view, there will be adaptation in which the eye and brain will strive to discount the color and see things more or less as normal. For example, tinted sunglasses will color the world, but, as adaptation takes place, the tint of the glass will tend to be disregarded. If colors such as red and orange *tend* to increase blood pressure, pulse rate, and other autonomic functions, the stimulation will be temporary, after which response may drop *below* normal. Conversely, if blue tends to cause retardation, later responses may rise *above* normal. *From these observations it is clear that physiological and psychological color reactions, to be actively maintained, require constant change and sequence. And this constant change is precisely what will help to counteract sensory deprivation.*

COLOR SELECTION

Among light colors this writer prefers such tints as ivory, peach, pink, yellow, pale green, aqua—but not pale blue, which tends to create a cold and bleak look. Reflections below sixty percent are proposed to avoid the possibility of glare. Purples and violets (like light blue) are not advised, because of their symbolic associations with mourning and because their afterimages will cast a yellow-green pallor over an interior or the persons in it. Highly recommended are medium-deep accent colors such as coral, orange, gold, terra cotta, green, turquoise, and *medium or deep* blue. (Munsell notations for the colors listed above are given in the box that accompanies this chapter.)

Recommended colors for interiors where groups of persons are assembled or confined and where comfort and efficiency are to be assured. Notations are Munsell's.

> white, off-white 5Y 9/1
> (for ceilings)
>
> suntan beige 5YR 8/2
> (sequence color for walls)
>
> *light colors*
> peach 7.5YR 8/4
> pink 10R 8/4
> yellow 2.5Y 8.5/4
> pale green 10GY 8/2
> aqua 7.5BG 8/2
>
> *accent colors*
> coral 7.5R 6/10
> orange 5YR 6/10
> gold 2.5Y 6/8
> terra cotta 5R 5/6
> green 5GY 5/4
> turquoise 7.5BG 5/6
> blue 10B 5/6

END-WALL TREATMENTS

Great success has followed the use of white or off-white for ceilings and light or medium-light colors for floors and furnishings or equipment. A sequence color, such as beige or a suntan flesh tone, is specified for general wall areas. Medium or medium-deep accent colors, listed separately, are applied to end walls (but not to window walls). The warmer colors may be used for south or east exposures, rest and recreation areas, food service. The cooler colors may be used for work spaces. Monotony should be avoided. Treat the eyes and human moods to moderate variety. Sensory deprivation will be conquered, and the joy of color will keep spirits high—with no danger of visual, physical, mental, or emotional strain.

COLOR AND SAFETY

To keep people alert in areas where they may be exposed to hazards, color has had widespread and highly practical use. While this application only indirectly concerns sensory deprivation, it does serve a rational purpose in industry where indifference or monotony may cause attention to flag and where as a consequence there may be danger to life and limb.

In 1943 this writer, working in conjunction with the industrial-finishes division of the Du Pont Company, drew together a number of safety practices related to color and organized a code that was endorsed by the National Safety Council in 1944. The code was introduced in a big way in 1948 by the U.S. Navy in a manual prepared by this writer. It was partly accepted by the American National Standards Institute in 1945 and more fully in 1953. In time it became a worldwide code recommended by the International Organization for Standardization. The safety color code is now mandatory in the United States by a 1970 act of Congress, the Occupational Safety and Health Act (called OSHA), designed "To assure safe and healthful working conditions for working man and woman."

Here are the features of the code. Red is used for fire protection, fire-alarm boxes, fire extinguishers, fire hydrants and hose connections, sprinkler lines, fire-fighting equipment. Orange is used for acute hazards. It is painted along cutting edges, along exposed gears and pulleys, near or on saws, grinding wheels, sanders, routers, drills, shears, and planers. It is further applied to call attention to hot pipes, exposed electric wires or rails, and emergency control boxes on hazardous machinery. Yellow or yellow and black bands or stripes are applied to mark stumbling or falling hazards, low beams, obstructions, the edges of pits and platforms, railings around hazardous areas. It is also proper for road equipment, tractors, cranes, forklift trucks, and any vehicle operating in industrial areas. Blue has special applications in signs or symbols to mark equipment that should not be operated without permission: boilers, tanks, ovens, dryers, kilns, elevators. It is also standard for electrical boxes and may be used for motors, generators, and welding gear. Green, the color of medicine, is used to identify first-aid devices such as medicine and first-aid cabinets, stretcher boxes, cabinets for gas masks, controls for safety showers. Purple and yellow in a propeller symbol relate to extremely hazardous materials and devices associated with nuclear radiation. Black and white are reserved for mere instructional purposes, such as for signs. In addition to the Safety Color Code are codes for piping, compressed-gas cylinders, street and highway markings, airfield runway and danger markings, and other areas in need of distinction where color speaks a universal language, free of any need for literacy.

PSYCHIC LIGHTING

Color as used today is often bland, sweet, too much a pampered luxury. A contemporary preponderance of white walls is emotionally sterile and visually dangerous. A haphazard indulgence in bright accents—rugs, furniture, accessories—may be charming and all that, but it is largely meaningless. What may be done in a home is no one's business but the owner's and his decorator's, but, if the physiological and psychological needs of masses of people are to be served, colors should not be chosen on whim or impulse.

As modern civilization grows more complex, those responsible for planning environments will need to have a better understanding of people's psychic makeup. Other factors in addition to color need study, but at least its specification can avoid mere personal fancy. If people are to live in controlled environments, the physical conditions, such as light, heat, and food, can be directly and completely engineered—so should the psychological conditions.

In the future environments will be active, not static. Light and color effects, perhaps even the projection of patterns and scenes, will be monitored electronically for morning, noon, evening, and night, just as in nature. Some of the light will be programmed for physiological wellbeing, some for emotional stability. Natural day and night cycles and rhythms will keep man attuned to the harmonies with nature that have guided and controlled his existence over eons of time.

There is a new and highly potential promise of psychic lighting. The idea seems to have been inspired by the ingestion of LSD and other psychochemicals. One of its first manifestations is a "turned-on" world of brilliant, blazing, and flowing color. What is significant is that the *simulation* of mind-expanded states can be induced: one does not have to take hullucinogens. Turn up the lights, the colors, and the sounds, and people can be emotionally transported. Barriers are broken down, and somehow people exhibit less shyness and timidity. There is a good chance that psychic lighting may become one of the most important, functional, and rewarding contributions to the artificial environment of the future.

Psychic lighting has not come out of the laboratories of illuminating engineers. On the contrary, the psychedelic artist has scouted lighting equipment and made his own creative inventions. Scientists and artists now collaborate in an effort to see what can be done jointly. And there are new vehicles to exploit: polarized light, the laser beam, nuclear radiation.

The day is coming, and fast, when even the most conservative and austere environment may well be given more life and vitality through the introduction of psychic lighting in some form or another. In an office, factory, or school daylight sources plus some ultraviolet may be utilized for a good part of the day. For psychological and emotional reasons other light in other intensities and tints may be programmed: warm light in the morning, increased intensity and whiteness as the day progresses, "complexion" lighting at coffee breaks or during the lunch hour, pink or orange light at dusk.

For people with neurotic or even psychotic troubles "color therapy" of the psychedelic type may be prescribed as well as soothing music and other comforting sounds. As the practitioner of psychosomatic medicine knows only too well, a high percentage of human ailments, from asthma to ulcers, hives, stomach cramps, heart flutter, and shortness of breath, all too often originate in the mind. The afflicted mortal starts brooding over his misery and his condition worsens.

If light and color can help to save man from himself, draw him out of his despondency, and involve him agreeably in the world and with the people in it, then light and color by all means must have an essential place in the man-made environments of the future.

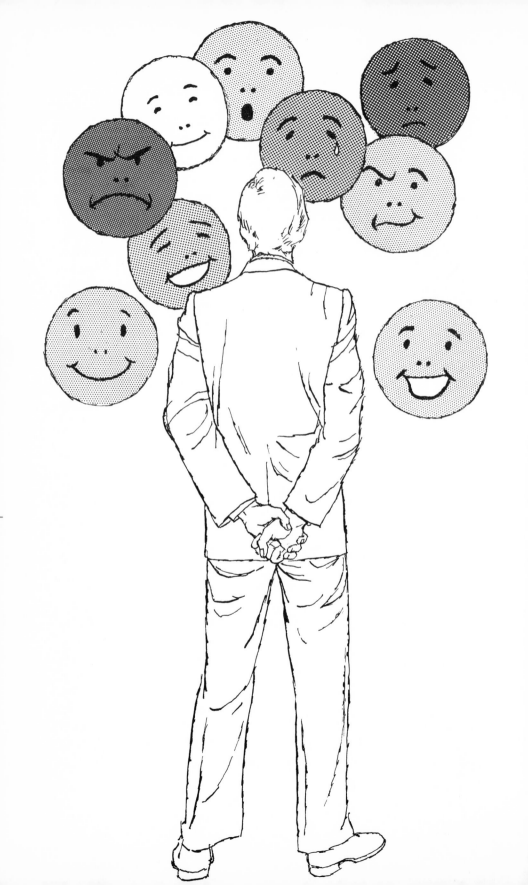

IX. Personal Color Preferences

Color preference as a clue to human personality is a controversial subject but by no means an unresearched or unstudied one. It is controversial for the simple reason that people are unalike. Even physiologically identical twins have different personalities. While there may be skeptics and disbelievers, the steady increase in mental illness across the land has encouraged new methods and theories of diagnosis, color among them. Although measurable facts can rarely be secured in the psychological sciences, broad and significant generalizations, even if empirically founded, are of interest to medical and psychiatric practice. As is described, certain generalizations that have a fully credible basis can be developed into tests and used as aids in delving into the mysteries of the human spirit, drawing from it simple and sometimes complex mental and emotional traits and peculiarities that may be by no means obvious in the appearance or demeanor of an individual. The great advantage is that admissions or statements of color preference by people are generally spontaneous and require little if any rational decision. People "love" color, so to speak, and will quite willingly participate in a color test. And in doing so they may lack suspicion of the test and may eagerly instead of reluctantly cooperate. Indeed, a negative attitude toward color or toward a color test will itself have significant meaning.

This chapter reviews diagnostic tests that involve color: Rorschach, the Color Pyramid test of Max Pfister, the Lüscher Color Test—and my own. Let me make clear that, while the Rorschach, Pfister, and Lüscher tests are scientific in purpose and concerned with mental dispositions or indispositions, my test is purely for entertainment and relates to people who consider themselves happily (or unhappily) normal. My research has been extensive, but it has been limited almost entirely to normal persons met under normal social and professional situations. The Rorschach test, not primarily involved with color, dates to 1921. (It was introduced to America in 1928.) My first color test, published in book form and signed with the pseudonym of Martin Lang, dates to 1940. The first

Lüscher test dates to 1947. The Pfister test dates to 1950. But let me begin at the beginning.

E. R. JAENSCH

The work of E. R. Jaensch is also mentioned in Chapter III in regard to eidetic imagery. Although his fascinating book on this subject dates to 1930, *after* Rorschach, one of Jaensch's observations can well serve as an introduction to the manifestations of color preference and personality—and at the same time posit a theory that may in part establish a visual and physiological basis for the whole subject.

Blond complexion types for the most part have a different attitude toward color than do brunets. In an attempt to explain this Jaensch mentions the difference between a predominance of "sunlight" in the more tropical regions of the world and of "skylight" in the more polar regions. As one travels from cold to hot climates, sunlight increases and skylight decreases. Intense light requires sun adaptation, or "red-sightedness," and this may be accompanied by pigmentation within the eye, probably for protection against excessive sunlight.

Red-sighted persons are typical brunets, such as the Latins. They are likely to have dark eyes, hair, and complexion. Their natural preference is for red and all warm hues, a predilection that may be far from spiritual in origin and is probably due to a physiological process of accommodation to long waves of light. Blonds, on the other hand, are "green-sighted" and may have a different pigmentation. They are the Nordic and Scandinavian types, with bluish eyes, light hair, and light complexion. Their preference is for blue and green.

To support Jaensch's theory, it is an observable fact that the deciding factor in color preference seems to be sunlight (or lack of it). Where sunlight is abundant, people are likely to show a preference for warm, vivid hues. Where there is relatively less sunlight, preference for cooler colors and softer tones will be found. I have found Jaensch's theory quite sound as to color preferences among Nordic and Latin types. Here, then, is a start upon which to build toward further refinements.

HERMANN RORSCHACH

Hermann Rorschach was born in 1884, the son of a Swiss art teacher. He studied medicine and took an early interest in mental illness. Though he died at the untimely age of 37, he created a series of psychodiagnostic test plates, famous and familiar today as inkblots that resemble butterflies. There were ten in all, five of which were black and white only, two black and red, and three in full color. They were meant to be shown to the mentally disturbed in the hopes of revealing signs of human neuroses, psychoses, and organic brain disorders.

Although the Rorschach test was disputed and criticized by some, it was also praised and accepted by others. It is still used today, and numerous books and articles have been written about it. It is fair to admit that facts and proofs regarding the Rorschach test may be set aside for assumptions and generalizations. Human personality is deceptive. No man, woman, or child is of one disposition or temperament at all times. Illness, circumstances, events may trouble the mind and cause no end of distortion. How, then, could Rorschach's inkblots be used?

Some persons were affected mostly by form, others by color. In interpreting the plates patients were asked to express their feelings, reactions, and associations. Some would think abstractly, whether plates were pretty or not, while others would think concretely and see things, birds, flowers. These responses required deliberation and ability to verbalize. But how about unspoken responses? Rorschach and his followers found another unique observation—to add to Jaensch's Nordics and Latins. As the plates were exposed, the researcher or diagnostician could watch the patient's facial and physical movements. Discovery: those who seemed well adjusted to life and the world and who evidently liked color—but who nevertheless were disturbed in some way—probably had tendencies toward manic-depression. Those who seemed distressed by color or appeared to reject it had tendencies toward schizophrenia. To bring in Carl Jung's reference to extroverts and introverts (people with outwardly directed interests as against those who are more introspective), it could be fairly stated that Latins, extroverts, and manic-depressives delighted in color, while to Nordics, introverts, and schizophrenics color was upsetting. In effect, there were positive and negative responses, and they were quite telling. (The reader may dispute this, but it does introduce some plausibility to the theme and justification of this chapter.)

Two Rorschach practitioners, Bruno Klopfer and Douglas Kelley, have this observation about the Rorschach test: "Probably the most important single sign of a neurotic reaction is color shock: all students of the method have found that neurotics invariably show such shock, and only a small percentage of normals and other types of pathology display it." Color acceptance or color rejection is thus revealing in a major way of outward or inward dispositions. It further suggests that there is psychological significance both in the individual colors that a person may *like* and in those that may be *disliked*. Rorschach and his followers have contributed much toward bringing reasonable order into the subject of this chapter.

To many neurotic persons, especially the schizophrenic (about sixty percent of hospitalized mental patients), color may represent an unwanted intrusion on their inner life. They simply don't like it or want it! With an alcoholic, for example, who may be an introvert while sober and an extrovert while inebriated, response to color may shift from disinterest to pleasure. Rorschach noted that reaction to color that might be more pronounced from time to time might be accepted as a measure of degree of dementia in epileptics. Color shock (rejection) was likely to be shown by schizophrenics, hysterics, and obsessive-compulsive human beings but rarely in manic-depressives. Persons suffering from neurasthenia (exhaustion, nervous breakdown) showed little reaction to color. If there were an emphasis on color over form, color might be considered "a deadly enemy threatening to break into the carefully isolated inner world of the patient, engulfing him in the dangerous whirlpools of reality relations which he cannot master." Severe depression might further be noted if the black-and-white cards were preferred to the color cards.

MAX PFISTER

Let me discuss briefly the work of Max Pfister. Though he published his *Color Pyramid Test* in 1950 (*after* Lüscher), it has not had the influence of Rorschach or Lüscher in the United States. In fact, Pfister's test has yet to become popular in the English language, although K. Warner Schaie of the University of South California has written of the test and of German literature devoted to it.

The Color Pyramid Test is meant to reveal "deviant personality characteristics." Patients are given black-and-white charts in which fifteen squares are arranged in the form of a pyramid, with five squares across the bottom and one square at the top. They are given equally small squares of color in twenty-four different hues and asked to put the color squares on a selection of pyramids. They were to respond on impulse, to express combinations that seemed harmonious and combinations that seemed ugly. Checks were then made by trained personnel.

To interpret some of Schaie's findings, persons who "scatter" the colors tend to be color-dominant, while those who "structure" the colors tend to be form-dominant. Attention is also paid to a liberal or restrained use of individual colors. A liberal use of red may indicate extroverted characteristics. Orange may suggest a desire to establish "good interpersonal relations." Yellow may suggest "determined personal relations." Green may suggest "symptoms of psychological disturbance." Blue might suggest the rational; purple, anxiety; white, tendencies toward schizophrenia. As Rorschach, Lüscher, and others (myself included) have noted, normal persons tend to prefer primary colors, while the disturbed may choose white, gray, brown, black.

MAX LÜSCHER

Rorschach, Pfister, and Lüscher are all Swiss, and their tests were originally published in the German language. Lüscher and this author have corresponded for several years. (One of Lüscher's students was associated with me for two years.) Lüscher's first test was issued in 1947 and included seventy-three colors on seven panels. A shorter test first appeared abroad in 1951. It was translated into English by Ian Scott and published in 1969. It has had a wide sale and has become quite popular in the United States. Lüscher has had his problems with the "factualists," as have Rorschach, Pfister (and myself).

While the Birren Color Analyst, described later in this chapter, is devoted to those persons, presumably normal, who wish to be entertained with fairly telling and revealing observations on their natures, the Lüscher Test in the American edition declares: "The Lüscher Color Test, despite the ease and speed with which it can be administered, is a 'deep' psychological test, developed for the use of psychiatrists, psychologists, physicians and those who are professionally involved with the conscious and unconscious characteristics and motivations of others. It is *NOT* a parlor game, and most emphatically it is not a weapon to be used in a general contest of one-upmanship." If Lüscher's book is meant for a doctor's office, my own is meant for anyone's drawing room!

The Lüscher Test in the short edition includes eight colors, which are described as orange-red, bright yellow, blue-green, dark blue, violet, brown, neutral gray, and black. (The Birren Analyst includes twelve colors.) In undertaking the Lüscher Test a person arranges the eight colors from left to right in order of preference—the ones he likes best at the left, and the ones he likes least (or dislikes) at the right. The book is then consulted. Interpretations are given of best-liked and least-liked hues, for pairs of colors, and for combinations of best-liked with least-liked. This adds up to some 320 brief diagnostic comments or interpretations. Some of them are quite concise. I strongly recommend Lüscher's book, however, with full appreciation that his purpose is a serious rather than a casual one. Let me now describe Lüscher's views on best-liked and least-liked colors. (For the meanings of pairs and combinations the book itself should be consulted.)

A preference for orange-red may indicate vital force, desire, action. The color is impulsive and sexual and may be picked as a first choice by persons who suffer physical and/or mental exhaustion. Those who dislike orange-red may lack vitality or be distressed by problems in their life.

Bright yellow is a favorable first choice, according to Lüscher. These people are intelligent, like innovations, and have great hopes and expectations. They seek happiness "in all its countless forms from sexual adventure to philosophies offering enlightenment and perfection." If yellow is disliked, there are indications of disappointment in life, isolation, suspicion.

Blue-green as a first choice, like the color itself, suggests the natural —constancy, permanence, perseverance. Security may be desired and change resisted. Rejection of blue-green may indicate anxiety, fear of loss of wealth or status, or failure.

Dark blue suggests accomplishment, steadiness, order, conditions of peace. Rejection of dark blue may signal personal rejection. This may lead to a desire to escape or to strange behavior.

Violet to Lüscher means "mystic union" (of red and blue), "enchantment, a dream made fact, or magical state in which wishes are fulfilled." Rejection of violet may signify that a person chooses to avoid close relationships, "either personal or professional."

Brown is physical, related to security and conservatism. It is rarely put in first place, and where it is, "dispossessed and rootless" souls may be encountered. Brown is often the least-liked of colors. This may be a good token of a desire to be individual and independent.

Neutral gray, like brown and black, is usually a last or near-last choice by most persons. Gray is "neither subject nor object, neither inner nor outer, neither tension nor relaxation . . . Grey is a Berlin Wall, an Iron Curtain." Those who place it first wish to live within walls, to be left alone. Rejection of gray may reveal boredom and a wish to participate in life rather than remain isolated.

Black is rarely chosen as a favorite color, and when it is, a person may be "in revolt against Fate." It occupies last place in the Lüscher test more often than any of the seven other colors. In the last position it suggests a determination "not to have to relinquish anything."

THE COLOR PREFERENCES OF CHILDREN

Much work has been done with the Lüscher Test both here and abroad, and an extensive literature, mostly in German, has been assembled. The test has of course been applied for diagnostic purposes in psychological and psychiatric realms. It also has been used professionally in rating among applicants for employment. It is apparent and true that pronounced character traits can be revealed merely from black-and-white charts that list a person's responses and without personal interviews. This may lead to practical shortcuts in judging and classifying large numbers of persons and to weeding out those with poor potential. If illiteracy or foreign-language difficulties are involved, the color test is one of the easiest and most desirable ones to take as against tests involving words.

Before detailing the principles and theories of the Birren Color Analyst here are some comments on the general significance of color preference and personality and on the color responses of children. In 1949 B. J. Kouwer of Holland wrote his book *Colors and Their Character*. Though Kouwer used words and no color samples or plates, he confidently wrote, "The fact that a certain relationship exists between character and color preference has become evident from so many experiments that further proof is hardly required." To him, "Color perception is not an act involving only the retina and 'consciousness' but the body as a totality." Like Jaensch and Rorschach, Kouwer noted that the qualities of warmth and coolness in color related to different temperaments. Warmth in color suggested contact with environment; coolness suggested withdrawal.

In 1947 a remarkable work in two volumes, *Painting and Personality*, was published by Rose H. Alschuler and La Berta Weiss Hattwick. It has since been reprinted in paperback by the University of Chicago Press and offers the best treatise on the color reactions of children yet known to me. Alschuler and Hattwick have been concerned with the recently developed profession and science of art psychotherapy, which is devoted to the study of human personality through art expression. Children are none too articulate. They have a natural love of color and respond spontaneously to it. Their responses are quite significant. Alschuler and Hattwick claimed that "Color more than any other single aspect of painting has been of particular value in offering clues to the nature and the degree of children's emotional life." The youngsters are more responsive to color than to form and will delight in it through sheer pleasure. As they grow older and become less impulsive, as they submit to discipline, color may lose some of its intrinsic appeal. Small children are likely to favor warm and luminous colors such as red, orange, pink, yellow. With these colors their inner feelings are released. Children who use cool colors, blue, green, may be more deliberate and less impetuous. Use of black, brown, or gray may reveal some inner troubles. Here are some pertinent comments on the meaning of individual colors to children.

Red, used freely, may show a simple and uninhibited love of life. Used defiantly, red may reveal hostility or a desire for affection.

Orange is the social color and indicates a good adaptation to life and society (a conclusion also reached by Henner Ertel and mentioned in Chapter IV).

A liberal use of yellow may suggest timidity or an unconscious need for adult supervision.

Green, as would be expected, was a token of balance. Those who use it freely tend "to show a perceptible lack of strong, overtly expressed emotions."

Blue may suggest conformity, willingness to obey and to control or suppress feelings.

Alschuler and Hattwick have observed that not many children seem to hold much interest in purple. This conclusion is not confirmed by other investigators. Lüscher, for example, reported a strong preference for violet among preadolescent school children. To this author use of purple or violet by the young (which he has rarely encountered) may reveal a naive effort to be sophisticated.

Brown, black, and gray are seldom favored by children. The anal character of Freud may be exposed if brown is smeared haphazardly, perhaps signifying defiance to an adult demand for vigorous personal hygiene and cleanliness. Black may be used for mere delineation or for outlines. If it is impulsively applied by children, defiance may be shown, or fear and anxiety may be exposed.

THE BIRREN COLOR ANALYST

As mentioned at the beginning of this chapter, my first book on color preference and personality, signed with the name of Martin Lang, was dated 1940. To my knowledge it was the first work to be devoted exclusively to the subject. My interest in this area began in the late 30s more or less by coincidence. I had prepared a series of abstract color studies that had the same design but featured the chief colors of the spectrum from red to orange, yellow, green, blue, violet, and purple. These were exhibited on the walls of my studio in a continuous row. I promptly noted that strong likes and dislikes were expressed by many visitors and friends, with the emphasis on color, since the studies were otherwise the same. I began to maintain files of references and to look up the findings of others (Rorschach, Jaensch). In a short time I built up a library of references and case histories. A series of small leaflets, *What is Your Favorite Color*, prepared for a client, was enthusiastically received. The Martin Lang book followed. My research gained both speed and volume. In 1952 I did a wholly new book, *Your Color and Your Self*, which sold abundantly, led to articles and reviews both here and in England, and to radio and television appearances. Further case studies came my way, and in 1962 I did a third book, *Color in Your World*. This was a paperback and had a printing of 90,000 copies. A fourth and completely revised edition has been published by Macmillan (1978). It presents newer data based on further research and case histories regarding the emotional significance of color preferences.

GENERAL RESPONSE TO COLOR

The publications just mentioned may be consulted by the reader. In this chapter I deal mostly with my own experiences, personal interviews, and how my conclusions as to the significance of individual colors have been reached. There is nothing fixed or academic: I claim merely that what people have to say about the colors that they like (and dislike) tells much about their characters. And if a wealth of data is assembled, remarkably accurate and revealing deductions may be drawn that, if they do not relate to all persons, definitely apply to the majority!

As to *general* response to color, it is wholly normal for human beings to like any and all colors. Rejection, skepticism, or outright denial of emotional content in color probably indicates a disturbed, frustrated, or unhappy mortal. Undue exuberance over color, however, may be a sign of mental confusion, a flighty soul, the person who flits from one fancy or diversion to another and has poor direction and self-poise. It is wise to bear in mind that color preferences may change over the years. If a person admits such a change, this may well signify that the character of the person has undergone change. This is more likely to be found among introverts than among extroverts.

There is a major division between extroverts, who like warm colors, and introverts, who like cool colors. To quote Dr. Maria Rickers-Ovsiankina: "Finally, Jaensch, quite independently, again reached the same dichotomy [as Rorschach] of red yellow versus blue green. He finds that all people can be grouped in a way similar to red-green color blind subjects, namely into those more sensitive to the warm end of the spectrum and those more sensitive to the cold end. The warm color dominant subjects are characterized by an intimate relation to the visually perceptible world. They are receptive and open to outside influences. They seem to submerge themselves rather readily in their social environment. Their emotional life is characterized by warm feelings, suggestibility, and strong affects. All mental functions are rapid and highly integrated with each other. In the subject-object relationship, the emphasis is on the object.

"The cold color dominant subjects in the Jaensch experiments have a detached 'split-off' attitude to the outside world. They find it difficult to adapt themselves to new circumstances and to express themselves freely. Emotionally they are cold and reserved. In the subject-object relationship, the emphasis is on the subject. In short, the warm color dominant subject is Jaensch's outwardly integrated type, the cold color dominant his inwardly integrated type." There is considerable truth in this, enough to accept the observation as "factual." As a further fact, persons with an open character and disposition are likely to prefer simple colors. Those who are more complex and discriminating may express greater subtlety of choice.

RED

The two most commonly preferred colors are red and blue, and they usually relate to persons with extroverted or introverted tendencies— naturally or by deliberate choice. There are differing red types. The first comes honestly to the color, with outwardly directed interests; he or she is impulsive, possibly athletic, sexy, quick to speak his mind—right or wrong. A salient feature of the true red type is to be given to emotional ups and downs, to blame others or the world for any of his or her vexations. Life is meant to be exciting and happy, and if it isn't, something must be wrong. There may be tendencies toward manic-depressive psychoses, so self-control needs to be cultivated.

The complementary red type (best observed in personal contacts) is the meek and timid person who may choose the color because it signifies the brave qualities that he or she lacks. Look for wish-fulfillment, for sublimation, for hidden desires to have the courage of red.

If there is dislike of red, which is fairly common, look for a person who has been frustrated, defeated in some way, bitter and angry because of unfulfilled longings. A happy or successful life has somehow been denied, and the person is distraught and probably ill mentally if not physically.

PINK

Following a radio program in an upper-middle-class area of Connecticut during which an interviewer questioned me about a series of hues telephone calls and letters asked why no reference had been made to pink. Follow-ups were undertaken by the radio announcer. Pink types for the most part were dilettantes. They lived in fairly wealthy neighborhoods, were well educated, indulged, protected. They were red souls who, because of their careful guardianship, hadn't the courage to choose the color in its full intensity. Pink may also signify recall of youth, gentility, affection. It may be an assumed or acquired preference by some who have had a rough time in life, who have been mistreated and who yearn for the tenderness of pink.

To dislike pink? No one of sound and admirable character should be upset by an innocuous color such as pink! Such a dislike would indicate annoyance with if not ire toward those who are pampered and indulged, the rich, the sophisticated, the vain.

ORANGE

Orange is the social color, cheerful, luminous, and warm rather than hot like red. It typifies the Irish character (orange is in the Irish flag), persons of enviable good cheer and with the unique ability to get along with anyone, rich or poor, brilliant or stupid, high or low. Orange personalities are friendly, have a ready smile and a quick wit, and are fluent if not profound in speech. They are good-natured and gregarious and do not like to be left alone. I have on rare occasions made the remark that the orange type may remain unmarried. If I have been wrong here more often than right, I have in a few instances been credited with amazing insight, for bachelors and spinsters have confessed to me—or friends have done so for them.

Orange is a color that is frequently disliked. There are those who "can't stand" the hail-fellow-well-met type, the politician, preacher, backslapper, quoter of trite aphorisms and poems. Life is a serious business. In several instances the disliker of orange has turned out to be a person, once flighty, who has made a determined effort to give up superficial ways for more sober application and diligence.

YELLOW

This color puts emphasis on the mental and spiritual and is chosen both by persons of good mind and intelligence—and by the mentally retarded (no humor intended). Marguerite Emery, in writing of the mentally disturbed, concluded, "Patients almost without exception who had regressed to, or had failed to progress beyond a markedly infantile level chose yellow." On the good side, yellow is often preferred by persons of above-average intelligence. It is of course associated with oriental philosophies. The yellow type likes innovation, originality, wisdom. This type tends to be introspective, discriminating, and high-minded and serious-minded about the world and the talented people in it.

Yellow in the western world has symbolized cowardice, prejudice, persecution. Some may dislike the color for this fair reason. It may appeal to troubled minds, to those who consciously or unconsciously disdain all that is intellectually involved or complex. This may be a mere defense against a person's own lack of mental stability.

YELLOW-GREEN

A discussion of this color has not been given much space in my books, as a preference for it has rarely been expressed to me. From the few cases in my experience I would conclude that the yellow-green type is perceptive, leads an inner life, but resents being looked upon as a recluse. There is a desire to win admiration for good qualities of mind and demeanor but difficulty in meeting with others because of an innate timidity and self-consciousness.

A dislike of yellow-green may indicate racial and social prejudice, a disdain of people because of religion, color, nationality.

GREEN

Green is perhaps the most American of colors. It is symbolic of nature, balance, normality. Those who prefer green almost invariably are socially well adjusted, civilized, conventional. They are persons who belong to clubs, take part in civic activities such as golf, cards, the theater. They are suburban, while orange types are urban. Here is perhaps an expression of Freud's oral character. Because the green types are constantly on the go and savor the good things of life, they are nearly always over-weight. They are the solid citizens of the world with easy manners and are not impulsive like red nor withdrawn like blue.

Dislike of green is encountered at times. It might indicate a degree of mental disturbance. The negative green type may resist social involve-ment, be upset by those who like the color, and otherwise lack the bal-ance that green itself suggests. Such a person may lead a complex, often lonely existence—or just dislike the color for its prosaic qualities and the conventionality of those who prefer it.

BLUE-GREEN

Preference for blue-green was one of my most intriguing discoveries. There were those who would say quite definitely that they liked neither blue nor green but did like *blue-green*. I soon associated the type with Freud's narcissism—self-love. Here were mostly people who were sophisticated and discriminating, who had excellent taste, were well dressed, charmingly egocentric, sensitive, and refined. The significance of this became quite clear. Children, extroverts, the outwardly oriented liked simple colors, blue or green, without reservation. To be exacting about color and color variations revealed a fussy nature. As they were mature, conceited, vain, certain pronounced traits could be deduced as to blue-green types. They were probably sexually frigid (which goes with narcissism) and probably divorced (which so often happens to the ex-tremely fastidious and affected). I have had a far better-than-average record of being correct in this judgment.

Where a dislike of blue-green was met, though seldom, there was an ardent denunciation of conceit in others, an attitude of "I am as good as you are," or "who do you think you are!" But both the likers and the dis-likers of blue-green had one trait in common: both were sure to be self-centered, whether with grace or with gruffness.

BLUE

Blue is the color of conservatism, accomplishment, devotion, delibera-tion, introspection. It therefore goes with people who succeed through application, those who know how to earn money, make the right connec-tions in life, and seldom do anything impulsive. They probably have a strong sex drive but one that is subject to careful control and manipulation. They make able executives and golfers, and they usually dwell in neighborhoods where other blue lovers are to be found. They are politically reactionary, and if by chance they mention a preference for *dark* blue, they are ultrareactionary. Being rational, they often look upon themselves and upon their life as exemplary, which it may not be. Blue types are cautious, steady, often admirable, and generally quite conscious of these virtues.

There is also the complementary blue type, the compulsive person who longs for the equanimity of blue. Blue is the Virgin Mary's color, mother, protector, full of love and patience. Impetuous Italians and Spaniards have at times expressed this preference for blue despite their red natures. They thus confess an inner desire for the benign life that has been denied them or that they have attempted to achieve for themselves.

A dislike for blue may signal revolt, guilt, a sense of failure, anger over the accomplishments of others who may not have expended the hard effort of the blue hater. Success in others may be resented—they have had the good breaks and good luck. There is perhaps weariness from having labored hard with little reward. In effect, a dislike of blue is something to regret, for it may lead to great unhappiness if not neurotic behavior.

PURPLE AND VIOLET

Purple and violet are subtle colors and are usually looked upon as elegant by the average person. Purple may be liked on the one hand by artists and persons of cultural bent and on the other as an affectation—i.e., lavender and old lace. On its good side, those who choose purple as a favorite color are usually sensitive and have above-average taste. While vanity may be involved, the purple lovers have unusual endowments, are fond of all the arts, of philosophy, the ballet, symphony, and other such refined pursuits. They may be temperamental but easy to live with if one is accepted by them. They carefully avoid the more sordid and vulgar aspects of life and have high ideals for themselves and for everyone else—but to their standards. As a side comment, some who say that they like purple may be lying and putting on an act: they may be anything but cultured and refined and only impertinent.

Those who dislike purple are enemies of pretense, vanity, conceit and will readily disparage things cultural, which to them may be purely artificial. People should be genuine and should not put aside the mundane and humble aspects of life. To those who dislike purple there is difficulty in separating spiritual qualities in others from that which is worldly. To them a blend of the two seems impossible.

BROWN

Brown is a color of the earth and is preferred by persons who have homespun qualities. They are sturdy, reliable, shrewd, parsimonious, look old when they are young and young when they are old. Here is conservatism in the extreme, a sense of duty and responsibility that may lead to paranoid tendencies. Being forever rational, those who are fond of brown may resent anything flighty in others but yet may be attracted to flightiness. They sit in the bleachers and seldom take an active part on the playing field.

More persons dislike brown than like it. In fact, brown is often preferred by the mentally troubled than by those who are at peace with themselves. What may be revealed in a distaste for brown is impatience with what is dull and boring. This might mean country life as against the excitement of the big city. Brown is very easy to dislike. For the most part, a negative and antagonistic attitude toward it is a good trait in anyone—and the same applies to antagonism toward white, gray, and black.

WHITE, GRAY, AND BLACK

White is not in the Lüscher Test, nor did this writer include it in the first three of his books. Virtually no one ever singles out white as a *first* choice of heart. The color is bleak, emotionless, sterile. But white, gray, and black do figure largely in the responses of disturbed mortals. K. Warner Schaie, in discussing the pyramid test in which wide assortments of colors are placed on black-and-white charts, noted that incidence of the use of white by schizophrenic patients was 76.6 percent as against 29.1 percent for supposedly normal persons! So anyone who places white first perhaps needs psychiatric attention. It would be better to dislike white, but here again few persons are encountered who so express themselves.

A preference for gray almost always represents a deliberate and cultivated choice. The person seeks security, relief from any decided ups or downs. Perhaps the person has remade his character. Gray is sober and indicates a willingness to keep on an even keel, to be reasonable, agreeable, useful in a restrained way. To dislike gray is less likely than to be indifferent to it. It may be that the disliker is weary of an uneventful life or upset by a feeling of mediocrity within himself. There may be a yearning to get out of a gray cell or prison and share more of a hedonistic existence.

As to black, only the mentally troubled are usually fascinated by it, though there are exceptions. Some few persons may take to the color for its sophistication, but in this preference they may attempt to hide their truer natures. They may wish to appear mysterious, but this in itself may be obvious. People who dislike black are legion. Black is death, the color of despair. In virtually all cases such persons will avoid the subjects of illness or death, will acknowledge no birthdays and never admit their ages. They loathe inevitabilities and would hold to the present forever and ever if they could.

Bibliography

Abbott, Arthur G., *The Color of Life*, McGraw-Hill Book Co., New York, 1947.

Albers, Josef, *Interaction of Color,* Yale University Press, 1963.

Allen, Grant, *The Colour-Sense*, Trubner & Co., London, 1879.

Alschuler, Rose H. and La Berta Weiss Hatwick, *Painting and Personality*, University of Chicago, 1947.

Aristotle, works of, Volume VI, *Opuscula*, Clarendon Press, Oxford, 1913.

Ashton, Sheila M. and H. E. Bellchambers, "Illumination, Colour Rendering and Visual Clarity," *Transactions Illuminating Engineering*, Vol. 1, No. 4, 1969.

Babbitt, Edwin D., *The Principles of Light and Color* (1878), edited and annotated by Faber Birren, University Books, New Hyde Park, New York, 1967.

Bagnall, Oscar, *The Origin and Properties of the Human Aura,* E. P. Dutton & Co., New York, 1937.

Beare, John I., *Greek Theories of Elementary Cognition*, Clarendon Press, Oxford, 1906.

Beck, Jacob, *Surface Color Perception*, Cornell University Press, Ithaca, New York, 1972.

Birren, Faber, *Functional Color*, Crimson Press, New York, 1937.

Birren, Faber, *Monument to Color*, McFarlane Warde McFarlane, New York, 1938.

Birren, Faber, *The Story of Color*, Crimson Press, Westport, Connecticut, 1941.

Birren, Faber, "The Ophthalmic Aspects of Illumination and Color," *Transactions American Academy of Ophthalmology and Otolaryngology*, May/June 1948.

Birren, Faber, *Your Color and Your Self*, Prang Co., Sandusky, Ohio, 1952.

Birren, Faber, "An Organic Approach to Illumination and Color," *Transactions American Academy of Ophthalmology and Otolaryngology*, January/February 1952.

Birren, Faber, "The Emotional Significance of Color Preference," *American Journal of Occupational Therapy*, March/April 1952.

Birren, Faber, *New Horizons in Color*, Reinhold Publishing Corp., New York, 1955.

Birren, Faber, "Safety on the Highway: A Problem of Vision, Visibility and Color," *American Journal of Ophthalmology*, February 1957.

Birren, Faber, "The Effects of Color on the Human Organism," *American Journal of Occupational Therapy*, May/June 1959.

Birren, Faber, "The Problem of Colour in Schools," *School and College*, November 1960.

Birren, Faber, *Color, Form and Space,* Reinhold Publishing Corp., New York, 1961.

Birren, Faber, *Color Psychology and Color Therapy*, University Books, New Hyde Park, New York, 1961.

Birren, Faber, *Creative Color*, Reinhold Publishing Corp., New York, 1961.

Birren, Faber, "The Rational Approach to Colour in Hospitals," *The Hospital,* September 1961.

Birren, Faber, *Color in Your World,* Collier Books, New York, 1961, 1978.

Birren, Faber, *Color—A Survey in Words and Pictures,* University Books, New Hyde Park, New York, 1963.

Birren, Faber, *Color for Interiors,* Whitney Library of Design, New York, 1963.

Birren, Faber, *History of Color in Painting,* Van Nostrand Reinhold Co., New York, 1965.

Birren, Faber, "Color It Color," *Progressive Architecture*, September 1967.

Birren, Faber, *Light, Color and Environment*, Van Nostrand Reinhold Co., New York, 1969.

Birren, Faber, *Principles of Color,* Van Nostrand Reinhold Co., New York, 1969.

Birren, Faber, "Psychological Implications of Color and Illumination," *Illuminating Engineering*, May 1969.

Birren, Faber, "Color, Sound and Psychic Response," *Color Engineering*, May/June 1969.

Birren, Faber, "Color and the Visual Environment," *Color Engineering*, July/August 1971.

Birren, Faber, "Color and Man-Made Environments: The Significance of Light," *Journal American Institute of Architects*, August 1972.

Birren, Faber, "Color and Man-Made Environments: Reactions of Body and Eye," *Journal American Institute of Architects*, September 1972.

Birren, Faber, "Color and Man-Made Environments: Reactions of Mind and Emotion," *Journal American Institute of Architects*, October 1972.

Birren, Faber, "Color Preference as a Clue to Personality," *Art Psychotherapy*, Vol. 1, pp. 13–16, 1973.

Birren, Faber, "A Colorful Environment for the Mentally Disturbed," *Art Psychotherapy*, Vol. 1, pp. 255–259, 1973.

Birren, Faber, "Light: What May Be Good for the Body is not Necessarily Good for the Eye," *Lighting Design and Application*, July 1974.

Birren, Faber, *Color Perception in Art*, Van Nostrand Reinhold Co., New York, 1976.

Birren, Faber and Henry L. Logan, "The Agreeable Environment," *Progressive Architecture*, August 1960.

Bissonnette, T. H., "Experimental Modification of Breeding Cycles in Goats," *Physiological Zoology*, July 1941.

Blum, Harold Francis, *Photodynamic Action and Diseases Caused by Light*, Reinhold Publishing Corp., 1941.

Boring, Edwin G., *Sensation and Perception in the History of Experimental Psychology*, D. Appleton-Century, New York, 1941.

Boyle, Robert, *Experiments and Considerations Touching Colours*, printed for Henry Herringman, London, 1670.

Bragg, Sir William, *The Universe of Light*, Macmillan Co., New York, 1934.

Brewster, Sir David, *A Treatise on Optics*, Lea & Blanchard, Philadelphia, 1838.

Brown, Barbara B., *New Mind, New Body*, Harper & Row, New York, 1974.

Budge, E. A. Wallis, *Amulets and Superstitions*, Oxford University Press, London, 1930.

Budge, E. A. Wallis, *The Book of the Dead*, University Books, New Hyde Park, New York, 1960.

Burton, Sir Richard, *The Arabian Nights*, Modern Library, Random House, New York, 1920.

Byrd, R. E., *Alone*, Putnam, New York, 1938.

Cayce, Edgar, *Auras*, A. R. E. Press, Virginia Beach, Virginia, 1945.

Celsus on Medicine, C. Cox, London, 1831.

Chevreul, M., *The Principles of Harmony and Contrast of Colors* (1839), edited and annotated by Faber Birren, Reinhold Publishing Corp., New York, 1967.

Cohen, David, "Magnetic Fields of the Human Body," *Physics Today*, August 1975.

Colville, W. J., *Light and Color*, Macoy Publishing & Masonic Supply Co., New York, 1914.

Corlett, William Thomas, *The Medicine Man of the American Indian*, Charles C. Thomas, Springfield, Illinois, 1935.

Darwin, Charles, *The Descent of Man* (reprint of second edition, 1874), A. L. Burt Co., New York.

Da Vinci, Leonardo, A Treatise on Painting, George Bell & Sons, London, 1877.

Day, R. H., *Human Perception*, John Wiley & Sons, Sydney, Australia, 1969.

Dean, Stanley R., editor, *Psychiatry and Mysticism*, Nelson-Hall, Chicago, 1975.

De Givry, Grillot, *Witchcraft, Magic and Alchemy*, George G. Harrap & Co., Ltd., London, 1931.

Delacroix, Journal of, translated by Walter Pach, Covici, Friede, New York, 1937.

Deutsch, Felix, "Psycho-Physical Reactions of the Vascular System to Influence of Light and to Impression Gained through Light," *Folia Clinica Orientalia*, Vol. 1, Fasc. 3 and 4, 1937.

Dewan, Edmond M., "On the Possibility of a Perfect Rhythm Method of Birth Control by Periodic Light Stimulation," *American Journal Obstetrics and Gynecology*, December 1, 1967.

Diamond, Ivan et al, "Photodynamic Therapy of Malignant Tumors," talk at first annual meeting, American Society for Photobiology, June 13, 1973.

Duggar, Benjamin M., editor, *Biological Effects of Radiation*, McGraw-Hill Book Co., New York, 1936.

Dutt, Nripendra Kumar, *Origin and Growth of Caste in India*, Kegan Paul, Trench, Trubner & Co., London, 1931.

Eisenbud, Jule, *The World of Ted Serios*, William Morrow & Co., New York, 1967.

Ellinger, E. F., *The Biological Fundamentals of Radiation Therapy*, American Elsevier Publishing Co., New York, 1941.

Ellinger, E. F., *Medical Radiation Biology*, Charles C. Thomas, Springfield, Illinois, 1957.

Evans, Ralph M., *An Introduction to Color*, John Wiley & Sons, New York, 1948.

Evans, Ralph M., *The Perception of Color*, John Wiley & Sons, New York, 1974.

Eysenck, H. J., "A Critical and Experimental Study of Colour Preferences," *American Journal of Psychology*, July 1941.

Fergusson, James, *A History of Architecture in All Countries*, John Murray, London, 1893.

Ferree, C. E. and Gertrude Rand, "Lighting and the Hygiene of the Eye," *Archives of Ophthalmology*, July 1929.

Fox, William Sherwood, *The Mythology of all Races*, edited by Louis Herbert Gray, Marshall Jones Co., Boston, 1916.

Frazer, J. G., *The Golden Bough*, Macmillan, London, 1911.

Gerritsen, Frans, *Theory and Practice of Color*, Van Nostrand Reinhold Co., New York, 1975.

Gibson, James W., *The Perception of the Visual World*, Houghton Mifflin Co., Boston, 1950.

Giese, A. C., "The Photobiology of Blepharisma," talk at the third annual meeting, American Society for Photobiology, June 23, 1975.

Goethe, Johann Wolfgang von, *Theory of Colours (Farbenlehre)*, translated by Charles Lock Eastlake, John Murray, London, 1840.

Goldstein, Kurt, *The Organism*, American Book Co., New York, 1939.

Goldstein, Kurt, "Some Experimental Observations on the Influence of Color on the Function of the Organism," *Occupational Therapy and Rehabilitation*, June 1942.

Graves, Maitland, *The Art of Color and Design*, McGraw-Hill, New York, 1952.

Gregory, R. L., *Eye and Brain*, World University Library, New York, 1967.

Gregory, R. L., *The Intelligent Eye*, McGraw-Hill Book Co., New York, 1970.

Greulach, Victor A., *Science Digest*, March 1938.

Gruner, O. Cameron, *A Treatise on the Canon of Medicine of Avicenna*, Luzac & Co., London, 1930.

Guilford, J. P., "The Affective Value of Color as a Function of Hue, Tint, and Chroma," *Journal of Experimental Psychology*, June 1934.

Guilford, J. P., "A Study in Psychodynamics," *Psychometrika*, March 1939.

Haggard, Howard W., *Devils, Drugs and Doctors*, Harper & Bros., New York, 1929.

Hall, Manly P., *An Encyclopedic Outline of Masonic, Hermetic, Qabbalistic and Rosicrucian Symbolic Philosophy*, H. S. Crocker Co., San Francisco, 1928.

Heline, Corinne Dunklee, *Healing and Regeneration Through Color*, J. F. Rowny Press, Santa Barbara, 1945.

Heron, Woodburn, B. K. Doane, and T. H. Scott, "Visual Disturbances after Prolonged Perceptual Isolation," *Canadian Journal of Pschology*, March 1956.

Hessey, J. Dodson, *Colour in the Treatment of Disease*, Rider & Co., London (no date).

Howatt, R. Douglas, *Elements of Chromotherapy*, Actinic Press, London, 1938.

Huxley, Aldous, *The Doors of Perception*, Harper & Row, New York, 1963.

Iredell, C. E., *Colour and Cancer*, H. K. Lewis & Co., London, 1930.

Itten, Johannes, *The Art of Color*, Reinhold Publishing Corp., New York, 1961.

Itten, Johannes, *The Elements of Color*, foreword by Faber Birren, Van Nostrand Reinhold Co., New York, 1970.

Jacobsen, Egbert, *Basic Color*, Paul Theobald & Co., Chicago, 1948.

Jaensch, E. R., *Eidetic Imagery*, Kegan Paul, Trench, Trubner & Co., London, 1930.

Jarratt, Michael, "Phototherapy of Dye-Sensitized Herpes Virus," from abstract of talk at third annual meeting, American Society for Photobiology, Louisville, Kentucky, June 23, 1975.

Jarratt, Michael, "Photodynamic Inactivation of Herpes Simplex Virus," *Photochemistry and Photobiology*, April 1977.

Jayne, Walter Addison, *The Healing Gods of Ancient Civilizations*, Yale University Press, New Haven, 1925.

Jeans, Sir James, *The Mysterious Universe*, Macmillan, New York, 1932.

Jones, Tom Douglas, *The Art of Light and Color*, Van Nostrand Reinhold Co., New York, 1972.

Jung, Carl, *The Integration of the Personality*, Farrar & Rinehart, New York, 1939.

Jung, Carl, *Psychology and Alchemy*, Pantheon Books, Bollingen Series XX, New York, 1953.

Kandinsky, Wassily, *The Art of Spiritual Harmony*, translated by M. T. H. Sadler, Houghton Mifflin Co., Boston, 1914.

Kandinsky, Wassily, *Concerning the Spiritual in Art*, Wittenborn, Schultz, New York, 1947.

Katz, David, *The World of Colour*, Kegan Paul, Trench, Trubner & Co., London, 1935.

Katz, David, *Gestalt Psychology*, Ronald Press, New York, 1950.

Kilner, Walter J., *The Human Atmosphere*, Rebman Co., New York, 1911.

Klee, Paul, *The Thinking Eye,* George Wittenborn, New York, 1964.

Klein, Adrian Bernard, *Colour-Music, The Art of Light*, Crosby Lockwood & Son, London, 1930.

Klopfer, Bruno and Douglas McG. Kelley, *The Rorschach Technique*, World Book Co., Yonkers, New York, 1946.

Klüver, Heinrich, *Mescal and Mechanisms of Hallucinations*, University of Chicago Press, Chicago, 1966.

Knight, Richard Payne, *The Symbolical Language of Ancient Art and Mythology*, J. W. Bouton, New York, 1876.

Koffka, Kurt, *Principles of Gestalt Psychology*, Harcourt, Brace & Co., New York, 1935.

Köhler, Wolfgang, *Gestalt Psychology*, Liveright Publishing Corp., New York, 1947.

Koran of Mohammed, translated by George Sale, Regan Publishing Corp., Chicago, 1921.

Kouwer, B. J., *Colors and Their Character*, Martinus Nijhoff, The Hague, 1949.

Kovacs, Richard, *Electrotherapy and Light Therapy*, Lea & Febiger, Philadelphia, 1935.

Krippner, Stanley and Daniel Rubin, editors, *The Kirlian Aura*, Anchor Books, New York, 1974.

Kruithof, A. A., "Tubular Luminescence Lamp," *Philips Technical Review*, March 1941.

Laszlo, Josef, "Observations on Two New Artificial Lights for Reptile Displays," *International Zoo Yearbook*, 9:12–13, 1969.

Leadbeater, C. W., *Man Visible and Invisible*, Theosophical Publishing Society, London, 1920.

Leiderman, Herbert et al, "Sensory Deprivation," *Archives of Internal Medicine*, February 1958.

"Light and Medicine," *M.D.*, June 1976.

Logan, Henry L., "Outdoor Light for the Indoor Environment," *The Designer*, November 1970.

Loomis, W. F., "Rickets," *Scientific American*, December 1970.

Luckiesh, M., *The Science of Seeing*, D. Van Nostrand Co., New York, 1937.

Luckiesh, M., *Light, Vision, and Seeing*, D. Van Nostrand Co., New York, 1944.

Lüscher, Max, *The Lüscher Color Test*, Random House, New York, 1969.

Lutz, Frank E., "'Invisible' Colors of Flowers and Butterflies," *Natural History*, Vol. XXXIII, No. 6, November/December 1933.

Maclay, W. S. and E. Guttman, "Mescaline Hallucinations in Artists,"*Archives Neurology and Psychiatry*, January 1941.

Matthaei, Rupprecht, *Goethe's Color Theory*, Van Nostrand Reinhold Co., New York, 1970.

Melnick, Joseph L., "Herpes Virus Phototherapy: Should Studies be Continued?" *Infectious Diseases*, April 1976.

Mesmer, Franz Anton, *De Planetarum Influxu*, Paris, 1766.

Moss, Eric P., "Color Therapy," *Occupational Therapy and Rehabilitation*, February 1942.

Moss, Thelma, *The Probability of the Impossible*, J. P. Tarcher, Inc., Los Angeles, 1974.

Munsell, A. H., *A Color Notation*, Munsell Color Co., Baltimore, 1926.

Munsell, A. H., *A Grammar of Color*, edited and annotated by Faber Birren, Van Nostrand Reinhold Co., New York, 1969.

Newton, Sir Isaac, *Opticks*, William Innys, London, 1730 (reprinted by G. Bell & Sons, London, 1931).

Ornstein, Robert E., *The Mind Field*, Grossman Publishers, New York, 1976.

Ostrander, Sheila and Lynn Schroeder, *Psychic Discoveries Behind the Iron Curtain*, Bantam Books, New York, 1970.

Ostrander, Sheila and Lynn Schroeder, *Handbook of Psi Discoveries*, Berkley Publishing Corp., New York, 1974.

Ostwald, Wilhelm, *The Color Primer*, edited and annotated by Faber Birren, Van Nostrand Reinhold Co., New York, 1969.

Ott, John N., *My Ivory Cellar*, Twentieth Century Press, Chicago, 1958.

Ott, John N., "Effects of Wavelengths of Light on Physiological Functions of Plants and Animals," *Illuminating Engineering*, April 1965.

Ott, John N. *Health and Light*, Devin-Adair Publishing Co., Greenwich, Connecticut, 1973.

Ousley, S. G. J., *The Power of the Rays*, L. N. Fowler & Co., London (no date).

Pancoast, N., *Blue and Red Light*, J. M. Stoddart & Co., Philadelphia, 1877.

Papyrus Ebers, translated from the German by Cyril P. Bryan, Geoffrey Bles, London, 1930.

Park, Willard Z., *Shamanism in Western North America*, Northwestern University, Evanston, Illinois, 1938.

Pleasonton, A. J., *Blue and Sun-Lights*, Claxton, Remsen & Haffelfinger, Philadelphia, 1876.

Pliny, *Natural History*, Henry G. Bohn, London, 1857.

Podolsky, Edward, *The Doctor Prescribes Colors*, National Library Press, New York, 1938.

Porter, Tom and Byron Mikellides, *Color for Architecture*, Van Nostrand Reinhold Co., New York, 1976.

Pressey, Sidney L., "The Influence of Color upon Mental and Motor Efficiency," *American Journal of Psychology*, July 1921.

Read, John, *Prelude to Chemistry*, Macmillan, New York, 1937.

Reynolds, Sir Joshua, *Discourses*, A. C. McClurg and Co., Chicago, 1891.

Rickers-Ovsiankina, Maria, "Some Theoretical Considerations Regarding the Rorschach Method," *Rorschach Research Exchange*, April 1943.

Romains, Jules, *Eyeless Sight*, G. P. Putnam's Sons, London, 1924.

Rood, Ogden, *Modern Chromatics* (1879), edited and annotated by Faber Birren, Van Nostrand Reinhold Co., New York, 1973.

Rothney, William B., "Rumination and Spasmus Nutans," *Hospital Practice*, September 1969.

Rubin, Herbert E. and Elias Katz, "Auroratone Films for the Treatment of Psychotic Depressions in an Army General Hospital," *Journal Clinical Psychology*, October 1946.

Russell, Edward D., *Design for Destiny*, Ballantine Books, New York, 1973.

Sander, G. G., *Colour in Health and Disease*, C. W. Daniel Co., London, 1926.

Schaie, K. Warner, "Scaling the Association between Colors and Mood-Tones," *American Journal of Psychology*, June 1961.

Schaie, K. Warner, "The Color Pyramid Test: a Nonverbal Technique for Personality Assessment," *Psychological Bulletin*, Vol. 60, No. 6, 1963.

Schaie, K. Warner, "On the Relation of Color and Personality," *Journal Projective Techniques and Personality Assessment*, Vol. 30, No. 6, 1966.

Scripture, E. W., *Thinking, Feeling, Doing*, Flood & Vincent, New York, 1895.

Sensory Deprivation, symposium held at Harvard Medical School, Harvard University Press, Cambridge, 1965.

Sheppard, Jr., J. J., *Human Color Perception*, Elsevier Publishing Co., New York, 1968.

Sisson, Thomas R. C. et al, "Blue Lamps in Phototherapy of Hyperbilirubenemia," *Journal Illumination Engineering Society*, January 1972.

Sisson, Thomas R. C. et al, "Phototherapy of Jaundice in Newborn Infant, II, Effect of Various Light Intensities," *Journal of Pediatrics*, July 1972.

Sisson, Thomas R. C., "The Role of Light in Human Environment," from abstract of talk at first annual meeting, American Society for Photobiology, Sarasota, Florida, June 12, 1973.

Sisson, Thomas R. C. et al, "Effect of Uncycled Light on Biologic Rhythm of Plasma Human Growth Hormone," from abstract of talk at third annual meeting, American Society for Photobiology, Louisville, Kentucky, June 23, 1975.

Sisson, Thomas R. C., "Photopharmacology: Light as Therapy," *Drug Therapy*, August 1976.

Smith, Kendric C., "The Science of Photobiology," *BioScience*, January 1974.

Solon, Leon V., "Polochromy," *Architectural Record*, New York, 1924.

Southall, James P. C., *Introduction to Physiological Optics*, Oxford University Press, New York, 1937.

Spalding, J. R., R. F. Archuleta, and L. N. Holland, "Influence of the Visible Color Spectrum on Activity in Mice," a study performed under the auspices of the U.S. Atomic Energy Commission.

Spiegelberg, Friedrich, *The Bible of the World*, Viking Press, New York, 1939.

Stevens, Ernest J., *Science of Colors and Rhythm*, published by the author, San Francisco, 1924.

Stratton, George Malcolm, *Theophrastus and the Greek Physiological Psychology before Aristotle*, George Allen & Unwin, London, 1917.

Tassman, I. S., *The Eye Manifestations of Internal Disease*, C. V. Mosby Co., St. Louis, 1946.

Thorington, Luke, L. Cunningham, and J. Parascondola, "The Illuminant in the Prevention and Phototherapy of Hyperbilirubinemia," *Illuminating Engineering*, April 1971.

Van der Veer, R. and G. Meijer, *Light and Plant Growth*, Philips Technical Library, Eindhoven, The Netherlands, 1959.

Vernon, M. D., *A Further Study of Visual Perception*, Cambridge University Press, London, 1954.

Vernon, M. D., *The Psychology of Perception*, Penguin Books, Harmondsworth, Middlesex, England, 1966.

Vogl, Thomas P., "Photomedicine," *Optics News*, Spring 1976.

Vollmer, Herman, "Studies on Biological Effect of Colored Light," *Archives Physical Therapy*, April 1938.

Walls, G. L., *The Vertebrate Eye*, Cranbrook Press, Bloomfield Hills, Michigan, 1942.

Watters, Harry, David Nowlis, and Edward C. Wortz, "Habitability Assessment Program (Tektite)," abstract, National Aeronautics and Space Administration, Huntsville, Alabama, 1971.

Werner, Heinz, *Comparative Psychology of Mental Development*, Follett Publishing Co., Chicago, 1948.

White, George Starr, *The Story of the Human Aura*, published by the author, Los Angeles, 1928.

Williams, C. A. S., *Outlines of Chinese Symbolism*, Customs College Press, Peiping, China, 1931.

Wilman, C. W., *Seeing and Perceiving*, Pergamon Press, London, 1966.

Woidich, Francis, *The Resonant Brain*, published by the author, McLean, Virginia, 1972.

Woolley, C. Leonard, *Ur of the Chaldees*, Charles Scribner's Sons, New York, 1930.

Wurtman, Richard J., "Biological Implications of Artificial Illumination," *Illuminating Engineering*, October 1968.

Wurtman, Richard J., "The Pineal and Endocrine Function," *Hospital Practice*, January 1969.

Wurtman, Richard J., "The Effects of Light on the Human Body," *Scientific American*, July 1975.

Zamkova, M. A. and E. I. Krivitskaya, "Effect of Irradiation by Ultraviolet Erythrine Lamps on the Working Ability of School Children," Pedagogical Institute, Leningrad, 1966.

Index

Vernon, M. D. 97, 99, 100
Vesalius 88
violet 14, 18, 19, 24, 29, 35, 36, 37, 40,
57, 58, 59, 60, 62, 65, 66, 67, 71, 74,
79, 80, 89, 93, 94, 105, 106, 115, 116,
124–125
vision
　colored 40–41
　human 34–35
Vogl, Thomas P. 94
Vollmer, Herman 23

Wagner, Richard 49
Walls, Gordon Lynn 18
Walton, William E. 66
Watters, Harry H. 101
Weiss, H. B. 18
white 1, 2, 3, 4, 5, 6, 8, 9, 10, 27, 31,
36, 38, 39, 41, 51, 54, 55, 56, 60, 62,
63, 64, 65, 71, 84, 86, 87, 88, 90, 105,
107, 108, 113, 114, 115, 117, 125–126

White, George Starr 73
White, Paul Dudley 78
Wilfred, Thomas 49
Williams, C. A. S. 3
Woidich, Francis 22
Woolley, C. Leonard 7, 8
world *see* color, of world
Wortz, Edward C. 101
Wurtman, Richard J. 13, 92

x rays 14, 15, 18, 88, 91

yellow 1, 2, 3, 4, 5, 6, 8, 9, 10, 14, 16,
18, 19, 24, 29, 35, 36, 37, 39, 40, 41,
45, 51, 54, 55, 56, 57, 59, 60, 62, 65,
66, 67, 71, 73, 74, 83, 84, 85, 86, 87,
89, 91, 94, 95, 105, 106, 107, 108, 115,
116, 117, 118, 119, 122

Zuckerman, Marvin 101